"The world is full of magic things, patiently waiting for our senses to grow sharper."

— W.B. Yeats

All Rights Reserved. No part of this publication may be reproduced in any form or by any means, including scanning, photocopying, or otherwise without prior written permission of the copyright holder.

Copyright © 2014 Elizabeth Ashley - The Secret Healer

Introduction

There is nothing worse than feeling poorly, is there? Stuffy nose, sore throat, headache, even period pain...and then you can't get to see the doctor for a week. Seven more days of misery ahead...it seems almost too much to bear!

Of course, the question is: are you brave enough to endure the joys of the surgery waiting room anyway? Welcome to the world's most successful breeding ground for germs. An old man in the corner hacks up a mucous laden cough, and the woman opposite seems positively riddled with sores. (Could that be leprosy? She certainly doesn't look good, does she?!) You can just sense bacteria marching towards you waving their placards of joy.

"Reduced immune system alert, chaps! All aboard, there's room for one more!!" That's it then. You might as well put up banners and balloons. They have declared open house and are intent on staying a while.

Interestingly enough, the doctor's likely to tell you not to be too quick to leap on the meds. Bugs are antibiotic resistant and our bodies are in drug weakened states. Our centrally heated houses, and air conditioned cars mean we no longer have immune systems that can put up good fights.

So, the medical fraternity are turning more and more to complementary medicine to find alternatives to shoving chemically engineered drugs into our systems all of the time. They encourage patients to find ways to improve their overall health on a day to day basis.

The days of *preventative* medicine are here.

Aromatherapy is a great place to start.

Essential oils ignite physiological changes to improve health beyond compare. They boost immune systems, balance hormones, stabilise blood pressure and even regulate appetite. They can help you to breathe more easily, stop your skin itching, soothe period pains and even settle your stomach. I've not even scratched the surface with that list, so it is wonderful you have searched to find out more.

On the day I write this though, there are 1,120 aromatherapy e-books listed on Amazon. By the time you read it, there will undoubtedly be more. It made me wonder what I could show you different to every other introductory guide available. What could I give you that none of the other books had to offer?

Well, before I answer, just indulge me for a moment...

Imagine you were walking through dense woodland on a crisp autumn day. Amongst the golden leaves you spy a rich, orange fungus glistening in the sun.

Let's you and me toss it in a pan and have it for dinner with lashings of parsley!!!

Go on! It should be OK, shouldn't it? Most mushrooms are safe to eat. Some of them are utterly delicious. What harm could it do to have just a wee taste?

Hesitant...?

I would be too, and despite the hype of the all the pages on the internet that is exactly the same caution you should be expressing about essential oils. Plant healing is wonderful in the hands of an expert, or even with a well read beginner...you simply have to know a few tricks of the trade.

The problem is, with the advent of the internet, not everyone writing about them has experience at their fingertips. And that's where problems can start.

Sprinkle the wrong oil in your bath and you may as well douse yourself with acid; some will irritate your skin that much. Fail to understand the capacity of an oil and a visit to the emergency room is not out of the question. Wrongly used, essential oils are very dangerous things. Without the right knowledge, choosing the best one is very difficult to do.

Make no mistake though; aromatherapy can do amazingly *beneficial* things too. Astonishing things, even. I have witnessed inconceivable changes in people's health. I have watched, gobsmacked, as symptoms have receded, right in front of my face. If you already love the scents of aromatherapy ...I am going to show you the *sense* of our art...the alchemy that turns plant essences into cold, hard, clinical tools.

First, let me be clear. I am not here to scare anyone. But the truth is, nothing magical only has a white side....I am simply going to raise my lantern so you can see dangers lurking in the dark. I want you to understand how to use your sorcery for the power of good in your lives...and I promise you, life is about to become a damn site more interesting. Because, those hands of yours have healing in them, and I am about to introduce you to the catalyst to make it flow.

Let *me* guide you through the woodland...because I know plant medicine very well. A hedge witch, perhaps? Who knows! What I am sure of, is I'm not touching that brightly coloured mushroom without seeing an expert one of them first. I'll even give him time to wash down a chilled glass of Chablis before that's going on my plate. I want to see the evidence of what it can do with my very own eyes.

I want to know he will put his money where his mouth is and back up his claims.

In this book, that is what I do.

If you want to learn about aromatherapy I am an excellent guide.

I have 21 years of professional experience and hold the Advanced Diploma of Aromatherapy. I know essential oils extremely well. Perhaps more importantly for you: I've no interest in airy fairy language, or over scientific jargon. I speak the language of flowers in exactly your dialect. I am easy to understand and (I hope) entertaining to read.

I'm here with a few of my qualified friends to show you some tricks of the trade. This is what I want to help *you* to do....

- Discover how to use a massive hundred different oils safely on yourself and on your loved ones.

- Uncover the chemistry that makes each essential oil magical in its own way.

- Become versed in the art of blending, creating scents that not only heal but smell incredible too.

- Save money on needless prescriptions and days lost off work feeling ill. For many conditions, aromatherapy can be a faster route to recovery than waiting for antibiotics from the doc.

- Get the hang of how to match oils to symptoms.

- Specialise in which oils you can use with no worries, and the ones to make your caution antenna twitch.

- Interpret safety data to double check your choices are right. (I reference the industry authority, *Essential Oil Safety*, by Robert Tisserand and Rodney Young 2013)

- Delight in the richness of just how magical essential oils can be.

You might think this is a long book at over 300 pages. In fact it is only the start. There are so many nuances, so diverse a capability, and so great a delight in aromatherapy…I just cannot show you all I want to, in the 30 or so pages other writers offer. So this book is considerably longer. It needs to be!

I want to give you ample opportunity to wallow in the silken mystery that is plant healing. But still, I suspect when you lift the lid of the aromatherapy cauldron and see how many possibilities are bubbling away....you may be hungry for more.

So if you like, consider *The Complete Guide to Clinical Aromatherapy & Essential Oils For The Physical Body* to be simply "Lesson 1" in your adventure, your induction into this arcane world.

Here, you learn how to treat the symptoms of illness. You gain a good understanding of what an essential oil is. I'll answer the questions, where did these strange elixirs come from, how are they made, how do we know what they can do? Step by step, I'll walk you through the stages of learning the properties of each oil, how to mix them together correctly for the strongest effects, and then I'll list ailments and their treatment oils for you to use.

For many, this will be instruction enough. But for those of you with more enquiring minds and a studious intellect, I have also included extra bonus material; monographs of six of the most interesting essential oils. These profiles detail the usage of lavender, rose, camomile, myrrh, geranium and tea tree - right back to the Ancient Egyptians and Australian aboriginal tribes, up to recent clinical trials undertaken into the oils by drug companies. You will gain unique insights into how our plants might be able to help conventional medicine find cures for disease; terminal and otherwise

To help you build further on your oils knowledge, I have included a chapter of recipe blends by other professional aromatherapists with their thoughts about the oils they have chosen to enable you see the nuances of essential oil healing even more clearly too. Not only, then, do you gain access to learner's tips in this book, I'd like to give you a sneaky peak into how some of the most advanced aromatherapists work too.

So you might consider this book to be your first aid kit, a sticking plaster, nothing more. In fact, to some extent I would call this essential oil therapy, rather than aromatherapy, because the therapy, itself, is capable of so much more.

Consider, a woman receives a late night visit from the police to be told her child has been killed. Tears and anguish bubble out, and then she violently vomits. No stomach bug caused this. This symptom came from emotional pain.

This example is an immediate response; the trauma racked her to the core. Sometimes, though, physical manifestations of our state of mind take longer to observe. Emotional state though, invariably underlies most of illness that racks the body.

Lesson 2, my book Aromatherapy for the *Essential Oils for the Mind Body Spirit - The Holistic Medicine of Clinical Aromatherapy* , investigates how the disease came about in the first place, and why certain things in our lives will trigger it to flare. In that book I teach you the steps to try to prevent symptoms coming back. I address how essential oils can affect emotions and in turn, encourage wellness to return. These are the essential oils for *Essential Oils for the Mind Body Spirit - The Holistic Medicine of Clinical Aromatherapy* . This is healing in its truest form.

But that's running before you can walk. Let's start by getting our heads around first aid....then you can learn the therapy.

So what about the price?

I am giving you over 300 pages and 25 years of aromatherapy experience entirely for little more than the cost of the printing!!! Other professional therapists have also generously given their experience because they feel passionately that aromatherapy can heal and people should know that.

I'll bet, though, some of you are looking for the catch.

Good for you!

My dad taught me there's no such thing as a free lunch, too.

There **is** something I'd like in return if you are happy to give it. **I'd love a review.** In fact I'd really like a thousand reviews, so if you fancy helping me out with that...great.

And, thank you very much for that too.

There is also a link at the back of the book for you to make a voluntary contribution to Cancer Research if you feel you would like to.

I'd also love you to go on to read the *Essential Oils for the Mind Body Spirit - The Holistic Medicine of Clinical Aromatherapy -* and perhaps even some of the manuals I have written for professional therapists too. You might also want to go on to collect other essential oil monographs as they each go on sale. But first I have to prove to you I understand what I am talking about!

So, come on then!

What are you waiting for....?

Turn the page to see if The Secret Healer delivers on her promises!

Table of Contents

Introduction 3
Table of Contents 14
Chapter 1 - The History of Aromatherapy................................... 28
Chapter 2 - What is aromatherapy?... 48
Chapter 3 - How do we know what an oil can do?........................54
    The chemistry of essential oils 56
        Terpenes.. 58
        Phenols.. 60
        Aldehydes 61
        Ketones.. 62
        Esters... 64
        Lactones and coumarins 66
    Botany of essential oils 67
        Chemotypes.. 69
        Headspace 71
    Extraction of essential oils..73
        Steam distillation...74
        Hydro distillation 74
        Rectification..75
        Cohobation...76
        Expression..76
        Solvent extraction 77

Enfleurage	78
Essential oil grading systems	78
Adulteration	83
Sustainability	84
Choosing Essential Oils	85
How to store essential oils	87
Chapter 4 How to use essential oils	**89**
How much oil to use	89
Carrier Oils	92
Almond Oil	95
Apricot Kernel	95
Borage	95
Calendula	95
Camellia	96
Coconut	96
Evening Primrose	97
Hazelnut	97
Jasmin	97
Jojoba	98
Peach Kernel	98
Rosehip	98
Sea Buckthorn	99
St John's Wort	99

- Tamanu 100
- Walnut 100
- Where to apply essential oils 100
- Ways to apply essential oils 102
  - Creams and lotions 102
  - Massage Oils 102
  - In the bath 102
  - Diffusers 103
  - Candles 103
  - Room sprays 104
  - Steam Inhalations 105
  - Compresses 106
  - Hot compress 106
  - Cold Compress 106
  - Homeopathic Dose 107
  - Neat 108
  - The Raindrop Technique 109
  - Neuro- auricular Technique (NAT) 110
  - Aromatouch 110
- Safety data 111
- Massage 115
  - Different types of massage 115
  - Benefits of Massage 115

The Physical Effects of Massage 117
Issues in the Tissues 120
Contraindications of massage 121
Massage Strokes 123
Hand positioning 125
Protection 126
Back Massage 127
Facial Massage 130
Chapter 5 How to blend essential oils 135
Chapter 6 The List of Ailments 139
    Abscess 140
    Aching muscles 140
    Acne 141
    Allergies 141
    Alopecia 141
    Aphrodisiac 141
    Appetite 141
    Arthritis 141
    Athletes foot 141
    Bed wetting 141
    Black heads 143
    Bladder infections 143
    Blood pressure 143

Breasts, sore 143

Broken skin 143

Bronchitis 143

Bruising 143

Burns 143

Candida 143

Cellulite 143

Chicken Pox 143

Circulation 144

Cold sores 144

Colds 144

Colic 144

Colitis 144

Concentration 144

Constipation 144

Cough 144

Cystitis 144

Dermatitis 144

Diarrhoea 144

Dry skin 145

Eczema 145

Fever 145

Fibromyalgia 145

Flatulence	145
Gingivitis	145
Gout	145
Haemorrhoids	145
Halitosis	145
Headaches	145
Herpes	146
Hyperactivity	146
IBS	147
Impotence	148
Infection	148
Insomnia	148
Neuralgia or nerve pain	148
Open pores	148
Pregnancy, Labour	148
Psoriasis	148
Rheumatism	149
Shingles	149
Sinusitis	149
Sore throats	149
Spots	150
Stretch marks	150
Thrush	151

Toothache 151

Varicose veins 151

Verruca 151

Warts 151

Worms 151

Chapter 7 Choosing Essential Oils 152

How to build an essential oils collection 152

The Essential Oils of the Physical Body 159

Agarwood 159

Angelica Root 161

Anise, Star 162

Anise 163

Basil, sweet 165

Basil, holy 166

Bay 167

Benzoin 168

Bergamot 169

Birch, white 170

Black Pepper 171

Bois de Rose 172

Cade 172

Cajuput 173

Calendula 174

Chamomile Maroc or Moroccan Chamomile 175
Chamomile Matricaria 176
Chamomile Roman 178
Cardamon 179
Caraway 180
Carrot Seed 181
Cassia 181
Catnip 182
Cedarwood Atlas 183
Cedarwood Virginian 184
Celery Seed 185
Cinnamon Bark 186
Cinnamon Leaf 186
Clary Sage 187
Clove Bud 188
Coriander Seed 189
Cumin 189
Cypress 190
Damiana 191
Dill 192
Elemi 192
Eucalyptus 193
Fennel 194

Fir, silver 196

Frankincense 197

Galangal 197

Galbanum..198

Geranium Egypt 199

Geranium Bourbon 200

Ginger...201

Gingergrass.. 202

Grapefruit.. 203

Helichrysum 204

Hinoki.. 205

Hyssop... 206

Inula 207

Jasmine 208

Juniper 209

Kanuka 210

Labdanum 211

Lavandin 212

Lavender 213

Lemon 214

Lemon Balm...216

Lemongrass..216

Lime..217

Linden Blossom 218
Litsea Cubeba 219
Mandarin 219
Manuka 221
Marjoram 222
Melissa 223
Myrrh 224
Myrtle 225
Neroli 225
Niaouli 226
Nutmeg 228
Olibanum 229
Orange, bitter 229
Orange, sweet 230
Oregano 230
Palma Rosa 231
Patchouli 232
Peppermint 232
Petitgrain 233
Pimento 234
Pine 235
Plai 236
Ravensara 237

Rose 238

Rosemary 239

Rosewood 241

Sage 241

Sandalwood 242

Spearmint 243

Spikenard 245

Tagetes 245

Tangerine 246

Tarragon 247

Tea Tree 247

Terebinth 248

Thyme 249

Tuberose 250

Valerian 251

Vertivert 252

Violet Leaf 253

Wintergreen 254

Yarrow 256

Ylang Ylang 256

Chapter 8 Oils for the systems 258

Respiratory System 258

Urinary system 258

Digestive System 259

Reproductive system 259

Aphrodisiac 259

Lymphatic system 259

Immunity and infection 260

Circulatory System 260

Muscular System and connective tissues 260

Skin 260

Nervous system – Physical 261

Mentally clearing 261

Chapter 9 - Essential Oil Recipes Designed by Professional Aromatherapists 262

Aphrodisiac Blend – By Annie Day of Heaven Scent Bliss .. 264

Depression blend by Dave Jackson of Cambridge Aromatherapy 267

Blend for ladies of that certain age... 269

by Clare Ella of Clare Ella Aromatherapy 269

Children's Cuts and Scrapes by Sharon Falsetto of Sedona Aromatherapy 274

Blend for Shingles by Jill Bruce of The Apothecary 275

Pregnancy and Labour Blend by Sue Mousley of SOME Training 277

Love Potion by Rebecca Brink of Serenity Thai Bodywork ... 281

Blend for Enhancing Self Esteem and Self Worth by Angela McKay 282

Migraine Compress by Erica Straus of Healing Essence Massage 284

James I Bandits Blend to Fight Infection – By Rebecca Totilo of Aromahut 286

Incision and Scar Healing Blend by Marcey DiCaro 288

Blend for Bruising by Natalie Miller from Aromatic Insights 289

Being Your Own Best Friend Blend – By Julie Nelson of Aromatique Essentials 291

Conclusion 296
Acknowledgments 300
Directory 303
Medical Glossary 327
About the Author 342
Other books in The Secret Healer Series 344
Works Cited 353

The history of aromatherapy....Where to begin?

Initially, when I started to write this book I had no intention of covering the history of aromatherapy. And yet, as the book has grown, my research has allowed me to speak to some of the most fascinating and generous people I could imagine, and I would like to share some of the things I have learnt with you.

Writing this particular book has been an adventure into the past. I have learned things I never dreamed I would. I have had correspondence from Egyptologists, botanists, mathematicians, chemists, and all because of these strange and enigmatic essences.

You are reading this bit first, but for me, writing this comes at the end of a long and extraordinary journey of discovery. I can see now, the history of plant medicine is so closely woven into how we use our oils, that by omitting the tale of how our magical healing came to be, in some ways I am concealing the enchantment from you. After all, plant medicine is the most fantastical, timeless, natural alchemy. It's only right you come to understand its complexities are anything but recently uncovered.

Chapter 1 - The History of Aromatherapy

The story, I feel begins in China, right back to the Neolithic Period. As the clouds of your imagination separate, perhaps you can discern the bitter sweet sharpness of resins being burned outside of a cave? The pungent smell pervades everything around it. The very earliest fossilised resins were found here, and on closer examination they were found to be charred. But why, I wonder? Could it be to cover the stench of rotting food, or perhaps as a way to speak with their gods? Maybe they had already discovered certain bugs or creatures would be repelled by its scent. As yet we do not know. Perhaps we never will.

It is difficult to surmise too, what these resins might have been. I am sure our Neolithic friend would have stared in fascination, just as we do today, as trees began to "cry" richly coloured tears from any breakages in their bark. Later evidence shows recipes of incense from ancient Chinese religious ceremonies dating to 2000BC contained cassia, cinnamon, styrax and sandalwood.

The lush lands of the Nile play a vitally important part in the history of plant medicine. We have gained more evidential information from their ancient civilisation than any other. Plant extracts were fundamental to their culture, being at the heart of their belief in the afterlife and their relationship with their gods. Frankincense and Myrrh resins were found in the tomb of

Tutankahmen. We now know these played a vital part in embalming mummies (I have written about this more in depth in the monograph about myrrh). Found with them, were jars of fragranced oils. Different to the essential oils we know today, the precious fragrances were absorbed into animal and vegetable fats. On opening the tomb in 1922, archaeologists were able to see one of the jars contained more than 450g of "resin" absorbed into animal fat. Over time the fat had created a wax seal over the opening of the jar, then had remained intact and airtight for thousands of years.

In the solidified wax, was a thumbprint, believed to have belonged to an intruder that had perhaps entered the tomb shortly after it had been sealed. Sadly, because the jars were opened by Carter's team the oil has now become oxidised and degraded. Had it been analysed in labs today, scientists would be able to match against biomarkers, not only to potentially more accurately identify the resin, but also to discern where it had originally grown. Resins and spices were traded extensively in and out of Egypt, many coming from the land of Punt but also from right across the Mediterranean.

In her book *Sacred Luxuries, Fragrance, Aromatherapy and Cosmetics of Ancient Egypt,* Lise Manniche tells of how a cargo ship sank on the Southern coast of Turkey, and settled on the seabed, 60 meters below, until it was discovered by Mehmed Çakir, a local sponge diver, in 1982. The wreck at Ulu Burun had lain there undiscovered for nearly 3,500 years. It was dated as being from around 1350BC by the discovery of a signet ring bearing the image of Nefertiti.

On investigation, the doomed ship contained almost one hundred jars of a resin identified as *Pistacia teribinthus*, which grows on Cyprus and *Pistacia atlantica*, native to Palestine. This is the resin from which we now have terebinth oil. It seems likely the ship would have travelled around the Mediterranean collecting resins and perhaps other plant extracts to bring to Egypt for further processing, for the Ancient Egyptians were masters of the art of oil extraction. They created magnificent oils revered by the entire ancient world.

A record by Dioscorides, the Roman doctor from around AD60, explains how the famous rose oil **Rhodinon** was prepared. As well as rose petals and oil, it also includes camel grass, which is thought to either be, what we know as lemongrass today, or possibly its cousin gingergrass. Both are now used as essential oils giving fresh, bright, aldehydic, citrus notes to blends.

Aspalathos is a well used ingredient in incense and perfume recipes of the period, but its exact identification still eludes us.

The Roman writer, Pliny, offers some clues as to what the plant might have been describing it as having a red coloured, strong smelling root. It had white, rose-like flowers and grew in Egypt and/or Rhodes. Some suggest this could possibly be a thorny bush called Camel Thorn, others offer that it might be some member of the *Convolvulus* family, which lead many to think it might be an ancient ancestor of our beloved rosewood, or bois de rose, amongst other botanical suggestions.

Sweet flag, still does not have a definitive identification either, but may possibly be *Acorus calamus L.*, an aromatic rush of the calamus of antiquity.

Lastly, rose perfume was blended with *alkhanet*, a dye that would best reflect the colour of the rose.

Rhodhion (Dioscorides)

Oil 9.220kg

1000 rose petals

Camel grass

2.494 kg aspalathos

(sweet flag)

Honey

Salt

Alkanet

"Bruise the camel grass, macerate with water, boil it stirring it up and down" and strain it into the oil. Throw in the "not wet" rose petals (i.e. free from dew), and, with your hands, anointed in honey, stir them "up and down" squeezing them gently every now and then. Leave them over night, then squeeze them out. Cast the strained roses into the labellum vessel, pour 3.772 kg of the thickened oil upon them. Strain again. Pour more oil unto the roses and strain again. This will be your second oil. You may repeat this a third and fourth time (to make a third and fourth oil), but you will anoint the vessel with honey each time. If you want to make a second transfusion (of each of these four oils) proceed with fresh dew free roses up until seven times, but no further. Always anoint your hands and the vessel with honey, stir up and down, and make sure that no juice is left with the oil, or else it will corrupt it."

Plant extracts, oils and resins were integral to the Ancient Egyptian way of life. Women beautified themselves with unguent cones strapped to their heads. The firm cakes of fats would soften in the heat of the day and they would become entirely engulfed in its heady fragrance. Interestingly, the scent would soon be lost to the wearer and only those around her would be able to smell it after a while. These luxuries would have been quite the status symbol.

Records show Cleopatra, renowned as much for her love of luxury as her beauty, on one occasion used 40 denariis worth of unguents to soften and perfume her hands. A denarii is thought to have equated to a day's wage and Pliny, later identifies that 40 denarii would have bought about a pound of unguent.

Sadly, Dr Manniche tells me, so far, she has been unable to find documented evidence of the beautiful queen ever actually having bathed in asses' milk. (I do hope she keeps on looking though, it is such a glorious image, don't you think?)

In 1874, George Ebers purchased a papyrus in Luxor, the site of the royal city of Thebes. This ancient parchment, dating to around 1550Bc offers us a valuable snapshot into health of the time as it lists herbs used to treat medical conditions. In total, it regales over 700 conditions with prescriptions.

As well as the plant data, it is interesting to see how the Ancient Egyptians considered anatomy. They recognised the heart, but thought that all blood, urine and tears stemmed from there, and so thus, so far had no conception of the kidneys. There is however an early understanding of mental health issues as the papyrus offers detailed sections about depression and also dementia. Some of the plants suggested are exactly the same as we aromatherapists might use today. If you do have an interest in this, I have placed a link to the full translation and commentary at buildyourownreality.com/resources

Plants and resins, in particular, played a vital role in the temple, purifying the air, offering sacrifice and opening a portal of communication, they believed, with their gods.

The finest, and most beloved resin, grew in Israel's sacred groves of Ein Gedi. The Balm of Gilead of the Old Testament seeped from the trees and was such a valuable commodity it became a political pawn in Cleopatra's power play for sovereignty.

In her book, Rebecca Totilo tells us...

"Josephus records when tensions were at their highest between Cleopatra and Herod the Great, Cleopatra contemplated seducing Herod to antagonise her husband Mark Anthony. On consideration she discovered a far more powerful play and encouraged Marc Anthony to give her the Balsam groves at Ein Gedi. The title deeds were handed over to the queen issuing a fierce blow to Israel.

After Cleopatra's death, Herod leased the groves back and the economy started to strengthen again. But peace was short lived because the temptation of the Balm of Gilead now had Rome in its grasp."

Other biblical references give many more clues as to how plants and herbs, in particular, were used in the period. Of particular interest is tithing, a kind of taxation system the Hebrews followed. They were obliged to tithe 10% of their produce and herbs to the temple each year. Herbs such as rue, mint and lavender were strewn on the temple floor and burned as part of their incenses.

Consider the functions this would have had. The temple was central to the Hebrew life. They ate there, met there and prayed there. In addition, they would sacrifice beasts to their God, the creature being slaughtered in the Temple. The stench, in the heat must have been hideous. It would have been full of flies and extremely unsanitary.

But then the devout stepped onto the herbs, crushing them beneath their feet, unleashing the essential oils of the plant. This sweeter space was far more acceptable for exchanges with their deity. The space was cleansed by the plants in every possible way, fragrantly, anti-biotically and spiritually.

This burning of herbs, inhalations and fumigation was a primary mode of "medical treatment" we see in the Ancient Egyptian texts too. More recently we have discovered ancient aboriginal medicine was likely to have been done in the same way. So far, this is the most effective way the ancient peoples can find of liberating the essential oil from the plant. Breathing in the fumes allowed the patient to enjoy the same benefits we do when we use a diffuser today.

Much of the information we know about this period, does not come from papyri as you would expect, but rather from Roman writers commentating on what they see happening in Egypt.

Pliny (AD 23-79) in particular, gives us a great deal of information in his work *Naturalis Historia*, the only one of his works to survive the temper of Vesuvius.

Galen too (AD 129-200) was a noted scholar of the period. He created many medicinal salves to repair wounds on Roman battle fields in particular. He utilises plants extensively and is attributed as having formulated the Cold Cream your gran might have stashed in her bathroom cupboard.

He was the most famous of the Roman doctors and a well-respected military surgeon. Many of the medical advancements of the period came from his studies. Because experimentation on human cadavers has been outlawed since AD150, he would dissect monkeys to try to understand more about anatomy and physiology of the body.

This man was a visionary in medicine, light years ahead of his time. His drive to understand the human body was unassailable. Other physicians mocked him and treated him with contempt when he refused to accept their surmission that illness came from mystical or divine sources. He was recorded as having argued "we must wait and observe". Two thousand years later, this might seem entirely obvious to us today. A doctor diagnoses and suggests the prognosis a disease might take. But we have history on our side; Galen was entirely revolutionary in his thinking. He was the very first person to understand "treatment of disease" as we know it.

I have a particular soft spot for Galen because he was interested in blood, like I am. (I should clarify this is because I have "problematic" blood rather than any vampiric tendencies you might get excited about!!!)

He was the first person to notice that blood going through the veins of the body was darker than those going through arteries. Now we know the ruby red comes from haemoglobin and the colour fades when oxygen leaves the blood.

Dioscorides too, was an avid collector and student of plants working under Nero. He created a massive five volumes of the *Materia Medica* which are vital reference texts.

Hippocrates, of course (he of Hippocratic Oath fame) was considered to be the "Father of Medicine". His work took Galen's hypotheses and built on top of them. He was able to ascertain *disease comes from something which is wrong within the body*. A vast number of plants are included in his writings. His works can be still be found in the library of Alexandria, now translated into Arabic.

As the mighty Roman Empire went into decline, their conquered world did too, both culturally and economically. The evidence of progress in medicine, herbal or otherwise, is lost in the dark ages to a certain extent.

But when Crusaders came back to Europe from the East in the 12th Century, it became clear learning had there, continued in earnest, most notably in the workshop of the great and famous Abu Ali Ibn Sina (980-1037 AD). So wise and revered was he, that his reputation went as far away as Rome, where in Latin he was referred to as Avicenna.

We know, now, that the Arabs had become enchanted with herbs and plants and whilst in the West, the knowledge languished somewhat, they had continued to research diligently.

Avicenna was a dedicated scholar, a philosopher and talented scientist. He wrote prolifically not only about his musings on health and the soul, but about plant medicine too. He enthusiastically toiled, creating beautifying elixirs and healing tonics. Whist we cannot be absolutely sure if he *discovered* distillation, his works contain the very first diagrams we have of the process, so it seems likely it may be so. It is thought the very first essential oil was made from rose petals, and that it was created, like all good creations, more by luck than judgement! This distillation is the process we still use to extract essential oils today.

Europe went into a frenzy when they discovered the incredible plants, resins, spices and oils Crusaders had brought from the Holy Lands. Suddenly, we can see evidence of trading between continents on a massive scale. Travellers began to use more herbal blends and they relished how many options of exotic ingredients were now available to them.

Clearly plant medicine was not restricted to these places, more our knowledge and experience is. Recent archaeological evidence from Cambodian World Heritage site Angkor Wat, demonstrates they, too, enjoyed a rich usage of medicinal plants. The diverse species grown within, would be taken to their temple for blessing and then were used to treat the inhabitants of the enormous city right up to 15th Century.

By the 15th century in Europe, essential oils were readily available in most apothecaries, but large houses created their own still rooms to extract elixirs from plants in their gardens. Evidence from this period can be found in plenty, but most notably we refer to Culpepper's Herbals.

During the so called "The Age Of Reason" of the 17th and early 18th centuries, scholars were mainly concerned with scientific and logical thinking and chemical substances took the place of plant medicine. But then, plant medicine takes an extraordinary turn in the late 18th and 19th centuries because scientists managed to identify that perhaps, it was not the plant per se, that made people better, but rather a single active ingredient that made it so. Here they began to look for ways to copy and synthesize the chemical component to use in conventional drug therapy. Quinine, digitalis and morphine were all formulated during this period, allowing many millions of people to be healed.

Now on the surface this may look like the beginning of a beautiful friendship between the two branches of complementary and orthodox medicine, but actually this is the very point where the two parted ways. Later, when we look at how an essential oil works, I shall explain why the two could no longer co-exist.

Scientists however, remained fascinated by essential oils. There was enthusiasm for trying to understand why a certain component of a plant might make it act in a certain way, but classification of the groups of chemicals was a monstrous task.

In 1910 Professor Otto Wallach of Göttingen University, stepped onto the podium to accept his Nobel Award for Chemistry for investigations into applications of terpenes of essential oils (alycilic compounds). His endeavours to categorise functional groups of compounds, which had so far taken him over 30 years to complete, continues to influence aromatherapy and research into plant medicine today.

In 1926, plant therapy, or phytotherapy as it was called by this time, took an extraordinary turn. A scientific paper by a French chemist was published about his findings whilst working in his family's perfumery business. Rénée Gattefosse severely burned his hand during an experiment, and looking for relief from the pain, he plunged his hand into the nearest vat of fluid available to him. Luckily (incredibly luckily, I always think when I discuss this...) the vat contained (not acid, but) lavender oil. He was shocked to find the lavender oil reduced the stinging almost instantaneously. He watched with interest, how much quicker his skin healed than he had expected and how no scarring was left behind. In a comparison of natural extracts and their synthetic copies, Gattefosse had been startled to find the antiseptic properties of natural extracts far outperformed those of their manufactured counterparts. From this paper a new term was born. *Aromatherapie* continues to be the name we call essential oil medicine today.

The touch paper had been lit and news of these remarkable new discoveries spread like wildfire across France. The twenties and thirties were a fertile land of experimentation. The cosmetic industry was transformed by skin care recipes by Marguerite Maury. A medical doctor from the University of Columbia, Andre Passebecq, set up "The School of Naturopathy, Vital Hygiene and Psychology". The centre ran for 40 years with Passebecq at the helm. "La Phyto-aromatherapie practique" was published by Marcel Bernadet. The works of these early healing pioneers form the foundation of the art we call aromatherapy today.

Make no mistake though, at this point aromatherapy is still very much fringe science. These were considered far-fetched ideas of an interested few. That is, until French doctor Jean Valnet came to hear of Gattefosse's claims and started to make studies of his own into the plants. His scientific objectivity allowed him to carry out experiments with a very analytical eye. He worked tirelessly throughout the rest of his life studying plants and recording his data. This is the first time we see plant medicine backed up by actual statistical evidence.

And then it all becomes a bit trippy...all a bit orange mushroom actually.

The experimentation of flower people of the sixties brought us a whole new hallucinogenic dimension of plants which had previously not been explored in the West. While some were simply mellowing in the groovy vibes, the esoteric movement began to explore connections between the mind, body and spirit. Aromatherapy gradually begins to become more complex. We begin to understand there is more to illness than the symptom and discover essential oils to be wonderful bridges between emotional, spiritual and physical health.

From this moment in aromatherapy's history, it is like a snowball running downhill. Alternative medicine seems to have been waiting for plant knowledge to catch up. We begin to understand the importance of the back and spine in health. We look at dietary needs and vitamin therapy. We find that essential oils can further improve the way Chinese medicine, acupressure and acupuncture can cleanse and detoxify the organs. Counselling and meditation begins to play a vital part in learning to control the mind and thus improve wellness.

In 1985, in the UK, the International Federation of Aromatherapy was formed and soon after the International Society of Professional Aromatherapists. This meant that even though, as such, we were not being legislated, there were bench marks of best practice being set in place. Structure and meaning was starting to take form for aromatherapy as a whole. It meant there was also a clear delineation between professional and amateur. This was a huge step forward for those who wanted to practice aromatherapy professionally.

In 1995 Robert Tisserand published *Essential Oil Safety: A Guide for Health Care Professionals* which gave us really detailed insights into not only the potentials of oils but also the pitfalls. In this book I reference his 2013 revised version of this.

In 1993, I became qualified! Aromatherapy looks a very different place to how it did then.

Now, everyone knows a little about aromatherapy, but not necessarily the full extent of what it can do. At the turn of the 21st Century you could buy essential oils off a supermarket shelf and every shampoo regaled the joys of tea tree contained within. In the scheme of things though, this glory day was short lived and, I suppose, in some ways, rightly so.

New guidelines by the Medicine's Controls Board and The Federal Drugs Agency, dictated that labelling of aromatherapy products had to change. Manufacturers were no longer able to blanket mark their product ranges as "Eczema Cream" or "Muscle Strain Lotion" because it was "Causing them to be drugs". Practice had to change. Conversations about how a certain product might help a certain patient could only be had after a detailed one to one consultation had taken place. This meant aromatherapy preparations could only be legally sold by a qualified aromatherapist.

But times are most definitely a-changing. With the advent of tighter legislation also comes a greater understanding and recognition of the public's desire to find more ways to become well. A 2009 report states that over a twelve month period the American public spent a breathtaking $34 million, in out of pocket expenses on complementary and alternative medicine. This acknowledgement has led to a significant change in our industry.

On June 5th 2013, Governor John Hickenlooper signed into law the Colorado Natural Health Consumer Protection Act (SB 13-215). This groundbreaking law means that access to natural medicine help is protected for all citizens of Colorado. (The number of Coloradans seeking out help from alternative and complementary practitioners in the 2009 report was deemed to be 1,500,000; no insignificant number!) The bill states that practitioners are now able to practice their medicine unimpeded as long as they stay inside of the confines of the bill. This disallows them from practicing surgery, puncturing the skin and other potentially dangerous practices. If you would like to read the bill of congress, please see buildyourownreality.com/resources

In 2014, knowledge of aromatherapy is easily accessible and simple to use. There are thousands upon thousands of gifted practitioners just waiting for your call. Essential oils are easy to obtain and are generally of a high quality. All that remains then is for you to learn what oils can do.

Step inside....I have much to show you.

Chapter 2 - What is aromatherapy?

Aromatherapy involves using concentrated essences of a plant to bring about change.

The word aromatherapy is somewhat misleading because it implies a patient gets better just because he/she smells an essential oil. This is only half the story. Sniffing an oil will alter mood, and in some ways *that is* medicine. If you're feeling tense and you relax, then this is most certainly therapeutic, but essential oils are capable of so much more.

They are made up of miniscule chemical molecules. It is believed each single drop of oil contains 40 million trillion molecules (that's 19 zeros!) That equates to 40,000 molecules for every single cell in your human body. These tiny molecules give essential oils their aroma. There are so many of them, that when you open the lid, they literally explode from the bottle dispersing into a room and filling it with their fragrance. This evaporation quality is what we call **volatility.**

These molecules are small enough to squeeze through the pores of your skin and enter your blood stream through the capillaries in the base of the dermal layers. From there, they circulate around the body to work in an incomprehensible number of different ways.

The molecules are also able to enter the body via your nose. Here the oils encounter nerves that send messages to an extraordinary mechanism called the limbic system. This part of the brain controls memories, moods, emotions, recognition and even learning. Inside the head, the brain has many structures protecting it from injury and contamination. The obvious one is the skull, but there are many more including what is called the Blood Brain Barrier (BBB).

The BBB does exactly what it says on the tin, it protects the brain from any germs or bacteria circulating in the blood. Scientists now believe, rather than being like a wall, stopping everything going through, the barrier acts like a sieve or a filter, if you like.

Very few things are able to pass this barrier. The molecules must be extremely tiny to permeate it. Meningitis bacteria are able to pass through, making it an extremely frightening condition. This tiny window of opportunity is exasperating for scientists, because it makes treating disease in the brain extremely difficult. Smaller molecules of chemotherapy, for instance, are able to permeate the barrier, but some of its larger molecules become blocked, making treating brain cancers with chemo impossible. They must be treated with smaller radiation, proton or cobalt therapies, amongst others.

To pass through the BBB, a molecule must be *inordinately* small, which of course those contained in essential oils are! Research shows that certain parts of essential oils *are* capable of passing through this barrier, opening up a new exciting arena for my friends in their lab coats. These magical oils come from a group called **Terpenes**, and we will look at them more closely in the chemistry section of the book.

For now, it is enough to know aromatherapy uses essential oils to make people better. It does this by administering oils in two ways, by inhalation and absorption through the skin.

Holistic Approach

This term refers to two facets of what we study in aromatherapy. We look at the whole of a person, that is not just the skin condition on their arm, but emotional factors that could trigger it, their diet and possible allergens causing it, how they feel about their situation in life, their work, their home etc. All of this will contribute to how their skin may flare up.

This is the basis of the rest of the books in this series. The skin is never red for no reason; something in the patient's life in the preceding days has caused it to happen. It has been irritated, maybe externally by washing powder and the like or internally by a factor we cannot see. For this reason complementary medicine works on the principle:

A person is made up of a Mind, a Body and a Spirit, rather than these being separate they are always influencing the others.

When you use an essential oil, it has **many benefits**. It can work on the physical problem, but it also has emotional and spiritual aspects too. Sometimes this can be wonderful, other times it can be less so. Rosemary, for instance is fantastic for improving memory, it is wonderful for easing nerve pain, it can reduce cholesterol, but if you suffer from epilepsy, it may cause you to fit. Ginger, the most deliciously warming oil is without compare in the bitter cold of winter. It stimulates the digestive system, kick starts circulation and encourages all of the other systems to work harder and faster too. Next morning though, you should also expect your bowels to be a lot looser, because digestion has been improved as a bi-product of the process!

Now to me this is where it becomes interesting. Traditional medicine, or as I call it allopathic medicine has always known plant medicine was useful; after all it predates their tablets and pills by many thousands of years. They have created many extraordinary drugs from components that started off their lives as plants.

Valium for instance comes from a beautiful tall weed I have growing in my faery garden. It originally came from the valerian plant whose bright pink flowers shade all of the ferns below it as they greet the sun in June. Interspersed between the valerian I also have fox gloves, the donor of the component of the heart medicine digitalis. Dotted around the garden, taking more and more hold every year are the poppies that first became opium, then morphed into morphine and less usefully also became heroin.

When the plant medicine is placed under a microscope it is easy to isolate exactly which part is having the desired effect (when you understand the chemistry it is even easier). Chemists separate off the active ingredient and synthesize it to make a chemical copy.

This is where we part ways because the moment you take the rest of the plant away, it becomes unstable. All of the other supporting ingredients keeping the constituent in check are gone. Remember I said an essential oil has many main effects? What do these synthetic copies have? Not main effects, rather side effects. Can you see the difference? Of course, the main outcome we can expect with the likes of valium and morphine (and to a lesser extent, digitalis) is addiction. This is a common side effect of plant created drugs when the active component is no longer regulated by other constituents.

Chapter 3 - How do we know what an oil can do?

In the early part of the 21st century, complementary medicine and allopathic medicine are no longer *us* and *them*. Whether either would admit it we have quite a symbiotic relationship. The guys in the labs don the safety goggles and see how oils will work on certain problems. But why did they think it would work anyway? For instance, why did a scientist go into his lab carrying a bottle of rose oil to test if it might help epilepsy? (Read the rose oil monograph to see if it does.)

Simple, they listened to the plant healers. They take information from our thoughts about what plants will help and go from there. But...where did we get it from? Sometimes the information is ancient and arcane, like the Ebers Papyrus. Dating from 1550BC, we can see healers already had ways to get rid of intestinal worms, calm people, improve appetite. The physicians at that time already *knew* just from watching their patients. After all, plants and foods were the only tools they had. Ayurveda too, has been helping us with plant wisdom for over 5000 years and legend has it this information was given to them divinely through the five sages.

We also have superb reference books like Essential Oil Safety Data Manual by Robert Tisserand that details which active components exist in each oil. This information must of course, have also originated from a lab and so the two disciplines continue to rely on each other.

Incidentally, what is fascinating is much of the information in the Ebers Papyrus and other medical information from those times is being vindicated by medical trials today. Thyme has been tested to assess its effects on internal parasites being contracted in Japan by a nation who eat raw fish. The result...the whole of the life in the petri dish was vanquished. Not a single parasite existed after the oil was left for just a few hours! How on earth did they know this back in the time of the Pharaohs? It's impossible to know.

The chemistry of essential oils

If like me, you were busy stuffing wooden splints in the plug holes of chemistry labs and putting condoms on gas taps when you should have been learning the basics of organic chemistry, you might be tempted to think this will be boring and difficult to follow. I can't argue for interest, but since I came out of school with the vibrant chemistry score of 18% you can expect simplicity! Actually, when you get past the dread of the thought of chemistry, your attention goes from boredom to scintillatingly electrical fascination, trust me…I'm *not* a doctor!

You will notice essential oil constituents tend to sound a bit like plants themselves because they are named after the plants they have been found in: geraniol, thymol, limonene etc

The main groups of constituents found in an essential oil are:

- Terpenes – usually ending in –ene as in myrcene or limonene

- Phenols – usually ending in –one or –in as in Quercetin, cyanidin

- Alcohols – usually ending in –ol as in ethanol

- Aldehydes – again, usually ending in –al or aldehyde as in formaldehyde

- Ketones – usually ending in –one as in thujone or pugelone

- Esters – usually ending in - yl then - ate as in linalyl acetate

- Lactones – usually end in olide or lactide

Essential oils, like anything living, are made up of carbon, hydrogen and oxygen molecules. Their main building block is called an isoprene (which is actually short for isoterpene). This is made up of 5 carbon units. Its chemical formula is:

$CH_2=C(CH_3)CH=CH_2$

Don't try to learn it, just know it is nothing more complex than a bit of carbon (C) and some hydrogen (H) molecules too.

The different categories of constituents depend on how these isoprenes are arranged into chains. How the carbon and hydrogen is put together will give the oil a chance to do different things.

Isoprene is an extremely volatile and colourless liquid, with a very low boiling point. If you remember, the volatility also means it evaporates very quickly too.

Terpenes

There are different types of terpenes within the family

Monoterpenes

Monoterpenes are found in almost all essential oils. They are made up of at least 10 carbon atoms and a double bond, so then, two isoprene chains linked securely together. The key actions of **monoterpenes** in an essential oil are **anti-inflammatory, antiseptic, antiviral** and **antibacterial**. They can also be very good decongestants. You will recognise lemon being in many cold medicines. Yes, it has high vitamin C content but it also has these other helpful qualities too. Vitamin C itself is too large to pass through the blood brain barrier and so it is the monoterpenes which actually make you *feel* better during the healing process whilst the vitamin C gets to work boosting the immune system.

Monoterpenes are very reactive to heat and light. Oils heavy on monoterpenes (like citrus oils) react to light and air very quickly. This is why you should not expect your grapefruit, lemon and orange oils to keep their strength for very long. After about 6 months the monoterpene content means they will have become oxidised and degraded...so frankly a bit rubbish for therapy!

Sesquiterpenes

These are almost magical in their **anti-inflammatory** qualities. They are made up of three isoprene chains, so have 15 carbon units and 24 hydrogen units. $C_{15}H_{24}$

Their effects are:

- ***anti-septic***
- ***anti-inflammatory***
- ***emotion and hormone balancing***

Sesquiterpenes are potentially the most important group of constituents because they carry oxygen molecules with them around the body to the brain. This extra shot of vitality gives the entire body, but especially the pituitary and pineal glands in the brain, a boost. If you struggle to imagine the effects, think of the giddiness champagne bubbles give you. Hormones are almost all influenced in some way by the pituitary gland so sesquiterpenes in an essential oil work a bit like you are switching the body up a gear.

There is a set of blue essential oils: spikenard, Chamomile matricaria and yarrow. These are all coloured by a sesquiterpene called azulene. It makes all these oils act like liquid anaesthetic is being stroked into your skin. It is very powerful indeed.

The interesting thing about this group is they have been found to actually reprogram errors written in DNA of the body. This has massive connotations for research into genetic influences of conditions such as migraine.

Phenols

Where terpenes used combinations of entire isoprene chains, phenols have side chains (incomplete sets of 5 carbon units in a chain). This makes them a bit edgier, a bit more unpredictable in type.

They are very strong ***antiseptic*** and ***antibacterial oils.*** They work very well as disinfectants. An oil high in phenols should only be used in low concentrations for short periods of time because they will irritate the skin or the mucous membranes of the body (linings inside the nose and lungs for instance). The body is not very good at ridding itself of phenols and so over time they accumulate as the liver is no longer able to cleanse them from the body. Clove and cinnamon are good examples of very cleansing oils with this fiercely sharp edge.

Aldehydes

These are the oils that smell refreshingly zingy and vibrant but are relaxing too. They are like a bright hazy day. Lemon balm (or as I call it Melissa), citronella, lemongrass are all good examples of oils where aldehydes are the predominate constituents. They have that sharp citrus edge that is bright, but they are very emotionally soothing too.

Their properties are:

- *anti-fungal*
- *anti-inflammatory*
- *disinfectant*
- *sedative yet uplifting*

This is a very unstable group meaning they can irritate the skin quite severely. They should only be used in dilutions of around 1%. Again, we have this potential oxidisation problem with this group. Oils with high aldehyde content will oxidise and go rancid very quickly, so prepare to replace your bottle about once every six months.

Ketones

This is quite a harsh group. Many of the oils on the International Federation of Aromatherapy hazardous list are there because of their high content of ketones. They are pervasive by nature, extremely penetrating and in large dilutions are simply too aggressive to the body.

In human physiology, ketones cause difficulties to diabetics. Normally our bodies can control the levels but when insulin is interrupted ketone levels get dangerously high. It makes sense then that a person with diabetes should veer away from large amounts or high concentrations of essential oils with high levels of ketone constituents.

Some ketones have neurotoxic properties too, so if a person is epileptic or has psychotic tendencies we stay away from even the smallest amounts of oils like rosemary, camphor, hyssop. High levels of pugelone in penny royal and thujone in sage have made both of these oils extremely difficult to use on women. Both oils cause very heavy bleeding, and use of pugelone in higher dilutions than 1% can be toxic to the liver and kidneys.

In lower concentrations though, some ketones can be extremely healing. In helichrysum oil for instance they are wonderful for healing scar tissue. In other oils they have excellent expectorant qualities that will reduce bronchial and chest congestion.

Most ketone components can be identified by the suffix *–one.*

Oils high in ketones are:

- Peppermint - Mentha x piperita
- Rosemary ct camphor - Rosmarinus officinalis ct camphor
- Rosemary ct verbenone - Rosmarinus officinalis ct verbenone/camphor
- Sage (Spanish) - Salvia lavandulifolia
- Spearmint - Mentha spicata
- Spike Lavender - Lavandula latifolia
- Turmeric - Curcuma longa
- Valerian (Root) - Valeriana officinalis
- Vetiver - Vetiveria zizanoides

Esters

When acids and alcohols combine, they form esters. I can remember making esters in a test tube at school and creating a product that smelled like pear drops. In fact all esters tend to have a fruity fragrance to them.

These are sedative and antispasmodic. They are also antifungal and anti- microbial.

Esters are easy to identify on a list of constituents as the acid part of their name ends in an –yl and the alcohol bit ends in – ate.

In nature, esters develop as the fruit ripens, hence the sweetness. A very common example occurs in lavender as Linalool matures into the ester linalyl acetate, so over time the alcohol morphs into an ester.

Mandarin oil is extremely rich in esters, but strangely its cousin tangerine has hardly any, this is because mandarin is distilled from the leaves of the tree, whereas tangerine is expressed from the peel of the fruit. This is interesting from several angles. Firstly, the properties of the oils are radically different from one another. Secondly, mandarin oil will last longer before there are concerns about oxidation and so might be a better oil to choose from an economical point of view. Lastly, when placed into a blend, although both oils are top notes (see blending) the mandarin fragrance unfolds slower and so lasts longer on the skin too.

One particular ester that appears in great abundance in some essential oils is methyl salicylate. This is a terpinoid ester which is very beneficial for muscle pain and is used in a great many liniments used for arthritis, rheumatism etc. Under laboratory conditions it has been found to be many times more potent than aspirin for its painkilling prowess. However, overdoses of levels of this ester cause convulsions, irritation to the intestines and gut if taken in too large a quantity. Poisoning from this constituent has a 50% mortality rate. Symptoms include nausea, vomiting, pulmonary oedema and pneumonia.

Just like aspirin too, methyl salicylate thins the blood and terrifyingly also makes the effects of blood thinning drugs far stronger, so patients on warfarin or heparin drugs are in more danger from this particular ester, because of the greatly increased chance of haemorrhage. When applied topically to damaged skin, its effects are enhanced considerably.

In the essential oil cassie, it is found in relatively weak dilutions of 11-19%

Chemical analysis shows sweet birch and wintergreen essential oils contain 98% methyl salicylate.

Lactones and coumarins

This is a small group and actually, most essential oils have extremely low concentrations of these. A lactone is a carbon ring with an ester inserted. Coumarins are a type of lactone. Chemically both of these act in very similar ways to ketones. They can be neuro-toxic and cause sensitization and irritation, but the risks of this are very low.

Lactones however are like snow ploughs careering through mucous, which is why Elecampane, also known as Inula is such an amazing oil for treating chest infections and bronchitis.

Coumarins, or specifically furocoumarins, actually play a far bigger part in perfumery than aromatherapy. There it is a useful ingredient. Coumarins are often taken from Tonka Bean. Here, it is a poisonous secretion produced naturally by the bean as a way to repel predators and insects. Its fragrance is like that of freshly mown hay. It is a very well sought after perfumery note and is responsible for the ovary clattering sensuality of fragrances like Shalimar. In 1953 the use of tonka beans as flavourings was banned in the USA as they were found to be damaging to the liver. Perfumery restrictions on the ingredient usage quickly followed. In Europe it is still widely available and small amounts of the bean added to drinking chocolate taste like heaven.

Because furocoumarins can cause phototoxicity (colour the skin in the sunshine) and can cause skin sensitisation, some oils to be used in aromatherapy are treated to remove them. A good example of this is bergamot fcf (furocoumarin free) where the bergaptene is removed making it less likely to make you blotchy in the summer time and easier for sensitive skins to use.

Botany of essential oils

You will notice essential oils are usually referred to by their Latin names. This is to avoid confusion between different species from the same plant family. We call these inter species variants: chemotypes.

The different parts of the name tell you different things about the plant. The correct name of this is binomial nomenclature - it means...two names.

The official classification of plants is called Taxonomy. They are separated into many orders, but as aromatherapists we are concerned with the family, the genus and the species (and very occasionally subspecies).

The classification takes many similar details about a plant and groups them together accordingly. Many botanists will tell you there are around 150 plant families where others will claim as many as 500. I would not like to comment except to say I would not like to have to learn them all, either way! The way to recognise the plant family is the name will end in **aceae**

A couple of examples:

Lamiaceae

This is a group you will be familiar with. It contains your lavenders, mints, oreganos, rosemary, basil, sage...the list goes on. So the criteria for classifying these all together are:

1. The petals of the flowers are fused together to make an upper and lower lip
2. All parts of the plant are aromatic
3. The leaves grow opposite each other and emerge at right angles to the preceding one

4. The stems are usually a cross section
5. The flowers grow in whorls and are bilaterally symmetrical

So where you thought these plants were dissimilar, you can see on closer inspection, actually they are not.

Asteraceae
This is the aster or daisy family. The chamomile belongs to this family. Their criteria are:

1. Herbaceous plants which grow from tap roots.
2. They have erect stems
3. The leaves grow alternate or opposite
4. The single flower heads are usually clusters of many tiny flowers.

A sunflower head is actually many flowers. Each petal is a strap shaped flower and on the ray disc in the centre are many flowers.

Chemotypes
Of everything about aromatherapy, this, to me is where the magic lives. A chemotype means a different variant of the species. Most commonly you might think of lavender, with all its

different colours and slightly different flowers. These are called different chemotypes.

Sometimes a plant will evolve to match the environment where it lives. Other times it might have been hybridized through human efforts. But when a new chemotype of a plant evolves, a new essential oil with different properties is also formed.

The most radical example I found of this was back in the early 1990s when I first trained. Croatian Lavender came onto the market. Its fragrance was sharp and cutting as if it had absorbed not only the chemicals of warfare into its soil, but its vibration and personality was more on edge, as if it were part of the war. By contrast Alpine Lavender was released onto the market at a similar time, harvested from way above pollution and noise, the oil was so gentle and serene it all most moved you to tears.

On a more mundane level, there are some chemotypes of everyday oils which are dangerous for use. Lavendula latifolia or spike lavender has high levels of ketones and can be neurotoxic in some cases. Lavendula stoechas is dangerous in pregnancy. If in doubt always aim for Lavendula angustifolia and grow your knowledge out from there.

Cinnamon is another oil to be watchful for. Cinnamon leaf is a fabulous antibacterial, but its counterpart Cinnamon bark is a particularly spiteful oil, to say the least.

Headspace

To the casual observer, essential oils may seem to be exact scent replicas of their host plants. It would make sense wouldn't it? In fact this is not so. In 1977 Drs Mookherjee, Trenkle, and Wilson discovered that the chemical constituents of the essential oil of a live plant were different to when it had been cut and thus changed its aroma profile.

Cleverly he attached a glass flask around a jasmine bloom and purged steam through it. After being cut benzyl acetate, once of the primary components that make up the heady fragrance of jasmine dropped from 60% of the chemical make up to just 40% of the oil.

Over the years scientists have been able to ascertain this may happen because the plant is trying to emit a defence mechanism. It is thought they gush essential oils to try to heal the damage our cutting has done and this imbalances the oil. For this reason, after being picked the plants are left for a couple of hours before undergoing extraction.

The oil profiles of many plants are also different when taken in the day and then taken again at night. Honeysuckle, as you would expect, alters, as does tuberose. What is fascinating is the essential oil is not simply stronger; the chemical composition actually changes as dusk approaches.

In tuberose, the limonene levels rise from 8% to 14% at nightfall but the methyl salicylate and alpha terpenol levels both drop radically, changing the scent of the plant.

What is interesting is when the headspace of different coloured roses is analysed, the chemical composition is slightly different in each one, leading to a slightly different fragrance. The primary chemical component of the luscious blood red damascena is nerol-geraniol, which is responsible for its sweet rosy scent. The same study analysed 5 different coloured roses to compare their aroma profiles. They compared blooms from Red Chrysler Imperial, White JFK, Red/Yellow Double Delight, Purple Intrigue, Otto of Rose Bulgarian.

Volatiles made up 30% of the "Bulgarian Otto" showing this constituent accounted for 30% of the oil, where as in Purple Intrigue it made up just 2.6%. In the other roses it showed no presence at all. Red Chrysler, by contrast, was bursting with citranellol which is a much lighter floral rose like fragrance. It also had quantities of 3,5-Dimethoxy toluene which is predominately found in roses of Chinese origin. The headspace of each rose was entirely different from rose to rose, even having completely unique chemicals contained in each.

Extraction of essential oils

There are many beginners' books with this information in so I shall make this section short to avoid probable repetition. We use the term essential oil to describe the essence of a plant that has been distilled. An oil obtained through any other method is called an absolute, or in the case of a carrier oil, a maceration.

There is a great deal of controversy over this point. Many say if the oil has not been distilled then it is not effective for therapy as it can have traces of adulterants in the oil. I do not subscribe to this school of thought. My own experiences have led me to see oils, extracted by many different means have therapeutic properties. The thought that you might not use the healing properties of a plant, just because it needs to be released through another method than steam distillation, seems very much like cutting your nose off to spite your face to me!

But, yes technically essential oils are extracted by steam or hydro distillation. If you are interested in finding out more about these processes, I would recommend seeking out books and videos by

Jeanne Rose and Marge Clarke who both have an enviable wealth of experience in this field.

Steam distillation

Plant matter is collected together in a vat, and then steam is purged through it at very high pressure and temperature. The heat releases the oils from the plant and they collect in the steam. The steam travels down a pipe to another vat where it is cooled. Because oil floats on water, you are left with two products. The essential oils floating on the top and beneath these is a water containing very dilute properties (and of course fragrance) of the plant as well. These are called floral waters or hydrolats. You are, no doubt, familiar with the most famous of these: rosewater.

This method is commonly used for twigs, leaves, roots and petals

Hydro distillation

Where steam distillation pushes steam up through the plant matter, hydro forces it down. It is very similar in process but will release greater volumes of oil from many plants.

Rectification

Sometimes you might see that an oil has been re-distilled or rectified. This might lead you to think the plant has gone through the process again, but this is not so.

Sometimes, after an oil has been distilled it may contain components which are not conducive to health, so the distillation process is interrupted and then repeated over again to remove the offending constituent. We call this fractional distillation.

It might be a certain oil may go through this several times. Ylang ylang for instance undergoes five re-distillations in order to remove the esters contained in the oil. In the final distillation the predominant constituents are sequiterpenes, but sadly these do not have the round, rich, sweet fragrance of the esters. The first distillation which has the finest and most exotic fragrance is called Ylang extra, then grades 1,2,3 become gradually softer. Which is the better one to use? Who can say, really? I suppose grade three is the safest but the least natural. You pays your money and you takes your pick, I think.

Camphor oil, too is extracted by fractional distillation because of toxic components. The first distillation yields essential oil and crude essential oil. This is then fractionalised and results in white, blue and brown camphor essential oils. We use white camphor in aromatherapy.

Cohobation

Sometimes steam distillation can separate important constituents of the oil off. In rose oil for instance, criminally, it actually removes phenyl ethyl, the part of the chemical make-up that gives us the distinctive fragrance. This is because the essential oil has partly bound itself to the water vapour. In cohobation, the remaining water is then distilled again isolating the active part and then this is re-added to the essential oil. This doubly distilled version of rose oil is called Rose Otto, and of course, is pricey, not only because the yield ratio of petals to oil is so small, but because this extraction process is so complex.

Expression

You could be forgiven for confusing lemon oil with lemon juice. In fact, citrus oils are taken from the exocarp or rind of the fruit. This is done by pressing the oils out in a process called *écuelle a piqué*. A machine puts hundreds of tiny pin pricks into the peel. It is then pressed very hard to release the oil.

The resulting liquid is then put into a centrifuge and spun very fast to separate off any contaminating water or extra products contained in the mix.

This is mostly used for citrus oils, which you will remember have a high concentration of monoterpenes. Luckily, this is a very inexpensive method of extraction, meaning replacing your lemon oil regularly is not as painful as replacing something like rose oil which has been extracted by a far more costly method.

There are some interesting anomalies to this. Whilst tangerine is expressed from the rind, mandarin is taken not from the fruit, but is steam distilled from the leaves which are far richer in oil.

Solvent extraction

In recent years this has become a very much more refined process producing a far superior product than historically was possible. In the past, solvents would be placed on plant matter to draw out the oil and then would be cleaned with alcohol. This method is usually used for extremely delicate flowers that will not readily give up their oil. Blooms like jasmine, honeysuckle, hyacinth and rose were all treated in this way. The problem was the solvent would leave behind a residue in the oil. Often the solvent itself may not be very pleasant, as in the case of hexane, for example.

More recently it has been possible to solvent extract using CO_2, which is an extremely clean process and produces a superior quality oil. Most chemical elements go through states of being solid, liquid and gas. CO2 however, has a moment where it is neither liquid or gas, we call this hypercritical. By taking the plant matter to a temperature where the CO2 is hypercritical it traps the essential oils. When the pressure is released the CO2 gas disperses and an extremely pure absolute is left behind.

Enfleurage

This is rarely used nowadays, but the romantic inside me is reluctant to leave it out. Most often, this method would be used to extract oils from roses and jasmine. Thousands upon thousands of petals would be laid on trays which had been smeared with vegetable oil. They would then be laid out in the sun for the rose oil to be absorbed into the vegetable fat. Time and time again, the trays would be changed to get more and more oil into the fat.

Then, like the other solvent extractions, the fat would be washed with an alcohol to separate the good from the bad. I love to imagine the heady scent there must have been, working with those trays. Sublime.

Essential oil grading systems

Useful as it would most certainly be, no such essential oil grading systems exist in aromatherapy today. Sadly, they are expensive and complicated to administrate, and we probably cannot expect to see any developments in this field any time soon.

There is often an inference that essential oils are ranked thus:

A – Therapeutic grade

B – Adulterated or synthetic

C – Perfume Oil

D – Floral water.

It can be easy for a newcomer to aromatherapy to become confused by this system, because often they notice the term "Therapeutic" and then imagine this is the benchmark they should be searching for. This is not so, because these terms are actually a tool created by multi level marketing (MLM) essential oil marketing companies to categorise their own oils. Look closely and you will notice Certified Pure Therapeutic Grade® is in fact a registered trade mark for a product of just one essential oil distributor. This means rather than being a benchmark, this is nothing more than a product name. The restrictions of trade marking dictate, no other company can use the term.

The grading system they use then, is not so much misleading, as arbitrary. The quality rating of their own oils, is commendable, but just because another company does not have the words "therapeutic grade" on the label, certainly does not make them inferior, (although there could be other factors that might, needless to say!) it simply means they belong to a different brand.

The International Standards Organisation or ISO, *does* have regulations about essential oil quality in place, which help us a little. This organisation offers awards to companies who can show transparency in their working practices. They look, not only at quality, but safety practices, potential hazards and how the company would deal with any, even how they source the components of their business or dispose of waste.

They have a variety of standards in place for different oils, ranging from how should you package an oil to the refractive index when the light touches it. It does not necessarily make a comment on the how well an oil will treat someone, but an award from them shows they can prove to another commercial buyer they are a reputable company, and have nothing to hide. If you are a saddo like me who gets excited by the science, the ISO benchmarks can be found at buildyourownreality.com/resources

AFNOR is a French, commercial organisation who do grade essential oils too, but only as a method of ensuring every oil that leaves France is superb, or at least very good. Both of these are very useful for us because they mean that pretty much all essential oils are of a certain (good) standard or the likes of AFNOR would not allow them to leave France because it might jeopardise the reputation of the country as one of the primary sources of essential oil.

But yes, to paraphrase George Orwell: Some oils are more equal than others; which brings us back to what some companies might class as Grade B.

The composition of an oil might make it superior for some reason; that is its actual chemical make-up. This composition could be different for a million reasons, perhaps the plant grew where there was no pollution and so it has a more benign structure. The oil may have been collected from plants all from one source, which would make it utterly sublime. Conversely, it may have been chemically altered to take away a certain troublesome constituent that irritates, reacts to sunlight, or even is carcinogenic.

So here is a question for you then:

If an essential oil producer changed the composition of an oil by taking out a component that was carcinogenic (and this does happen) is that oil now an inferior oil?

On the above grading system it is. It also implies you should have used the original oil to treat a patient.

Actually I am being a tad unfair, because there are no oils in the repertoire of the therapeutic grading system that would apply to the example I gave. But can you see the problems it creates?

In fact, changes in composition are not only not unusual, they are vital to keeping the essential oil industry alive. If a benchmark for an oil is it must have a certain level of esters, for instance, the producer needs to find ways to make the plant deliver that, otherwise how can he trade?

He might change the length of time he distils for, pick the plant at a different time of day, he might decide to water distil rather than steam because it gives a larger yield of most oils. He is changing his system to find a way to meet the industry benchmark of composition. Potentially this will yield a different composition to the first try, not better, not inferior, just different and closer to the industry standard.

Some methods can leave a residue, a contaminant. Most absolutes are contaminated in some manner and so this could imply they are adulterated in some way unless they were CO_2 extracted. The oil may also have been adulterated deliberately.

Adulteration

Sometimes essential oils may be adulterated with other oils. This process is called "cutting". Legally it must be declared on the labelling of the oil. Sometimes there is very good reason for it. Perhaps an essential oil might be prohibitively expensive on its own. *Melissa officinalis* or lemon balm, for instance, has an extremely low yield ratio. It takes a huge number of leaves to obtain a tiny amount of oil, meaning it costs a huge amount to produce. Often lemon grass or lemon verbena might be added to make the melissa go further. This is then called Melissa (Type).

The problem you have of course is the added oil changes, not only the scent of the oil, but also its properties too. You also need to consider that lemon grass has a higher chance of irritating the skin. Then, you must decide, with each purchase, if the trade off is worth it. In some patients, I will use Melissa type, perhaps for hayfever for instance, because there are no contraindications. But for a fragile little boy I treat with severe epilepsy, Melissa (True) would be the only oil I trust.

The same applies for rose oil. Again, it is a hideously expensive oil. I don't want to be throwing money down the plug hole every time I want to enjoy rose oil in my bath. I have a bottle of rose oil in 5% dilution with a rosehip carrier. That goes in the bath with me the expensive stuff goes in my face cream. It is an inferior product per se, but actually it is fitter for the use I have for it.

Definitely don't confuse perfume (or fragrance) oils with essential oils. They are synthetic copies with no properties other than they smell similar to the plant. They should always be labelled perfume oils, so reading the label is the only care you have to take here.

Bottom of the list is D – Floral waters. Again, they are placed at the bottom, presumably because they are so dilute, but actually they have more therapeutic use than a perfume oil.

Sustainability

We are lucky enough to live on a planet so magnificently resourced of natural medicine, yet paradoxically we farm these until there is nothing left! Sometimes restrictions have to be put on use of certain oils to protect them and allow them to re-establish themselves for future generations. Clearly this affects not only their availability, the quality of the oil, but also the price.

It is not always natural medicine that is the problem. Desire for beautiful furniture or perfumery fragrances can also be a factor, for example. In 1991, restrictions were placed on the trading of Brazilian Rosewood, *Dalbergia Nigra*, meaning only resources forested pre 1991 could now be used as commercial products. In fact, the dust from the wood caused skin and respiratory irritation. The oil we now term Rosewood is distilled from *Aniba rosaeodora*, an entirely separate genus, which has a similar scent but differing properties.

In India, Sandalwood trees have been so exhaustively forested for incenses, medicines and furniture that firm protocols have been put into place. Most commercial sandalwood is now imported from Australia.

In Japan, Hinoki wood is the most prized for construction of temples, theatres and high profile buildings. Its golden yellow surface exudes a classically Japanese scent. This is a lesser known oil in the west but is revered in Japan not only for its spiritual dimensions but its anti-inflammatory qualities too. Hinoki is now protected in Japan, but is also grown in Taiwan where a new sustainable essential oil industry is now emerging.

Choosing Essential Oils

Compare prices between websites.
Essential oil prices don't fluctuate very much, so if a price is too low, suspect some naughtiness is at play. Prices are generally very similar across the board.

Check your labels

Check your label shows things like country of origin and correct binomial nomenclature (remember how the first Latin name should be capitalised but not the second?). These show care and knowledge.

Extraction

Look to see what process was used to tease the oil from the plant. Expression is cheap so the oil should be too. CO_2 on a label means it has gone through a costly process and also you can expect the oil to be beautiful quality.

Where are they stored in the shop

If you go into the health food shop and they are close to the doors and windows you can guess they will be degraded. They will react to changes in light and temperature. Look for oils in a cool dark corner of the shop.

Manufacture dates

I am not a wasteful person. I have a freezer full of fruit suspended in animated decay. A sell by date on sausages doesn't worry me much but a short date code on a bottle of oil does, especially on a citrus oil. Make sure you have at least 5 months left on the code or frankly you have been conned.

Look for Value

Value will come from several areas: cost of extraction, how much yield a plant has, even its rarity will all contribute to its price. In the end though *for you*, value should come from only one area:

How much will I use it?

If you think you will only use it once in a blue moon, leave it on the shelf. Buy oils you will use a lot of in a short amount of time so they do not go out of date. Always remember:

Oils have many main effects. It is very rare you will not be able to find another better choice purchase to do the same job (albeit maybe not as effectively).

How to store essential oils

Essential oils should always be kept in dark bottles, in a cold dark place. I keep mine in those hobby cases the DIY stores sell to keep screws and bolts in, but I am thinking of investing in a beautiful wooden case.

Many essential oils are poisonous and equally as many are dermal irritants. I hate to think what might happen if you got some of certain oils in your eyes. They are not toys. Keep them out of reach of children.

One last pointer: always use glass bottles. I promise you every therapist has seen a pretty plastic bottle and tried to put a lovely mix in it. Essential oils eat through plastic and the prevailing mess on your shelves is really quite hideous.

Chapter 4 How to use essential oils

The most important thing to remember about essential oils is their potency. They are so strong, absorbing them through the skin is ample for the magic of their medicine to work.

They must be diluted in some way. It might be in a cream or lotion, a massage oil or even in a bath oil. There are a great number of sites on the internet saying their essential oils are safe to ingest orally. I would vehemently suggest you do not do this. Many oils have irritant properties that could burn the passage down to your gut. If you consider that together the large and small intestines measure about 28 ft in length, that could be a really painful episode.

To put it into context too, as professional aromatherapists, we have to take out insurances. If we prescribe this as a way of administering essential oils our policies are voided and no longer cover any accidents that could occur. It is that bad an idea. Please do not do it!!!

How much oil to use

This is kind of a how long is a piece of string question, but in my experience the answer is always…less than you think. It should really be one drop of essential oil to 25 drops of carrier, but frankly life is too short for any equation quite so fiddly.

The oils are very strong and trigger effects with very little help at all. Some, like clary sage and valerian become stupefying in large amounts. Others actually change from being relaxing to stimulating if you use too much. The old adage you were taught when cooking hold true here, you can always add a little bit more.

You will notice in the safety data for each oil, later in the book, sometimes there is a suggestion for a maximum dosage of particular oil. This is based on Essential Oil Safety Data from *Tisserand and Young*. It denotes the strongest dilution of an oil in trials that did not cause a skin reaction. This is useful advice if you are worried about a particular set of effects being too strong.

Helichrysum oil, for example is listed as no stronger than 0.5%. This means you will need 200 drops (10ml or about 2 tsp) of carrier to your one drop of essential oil.

When making a mix I would go for between 1-3 drops of an oil....three being if I think I need a sledgehammer. One or two will usually suffice. This also means you have room in your mix for far more oils.

In chapter 7, I have grouped the oils into systems to help you create an effect, rather than a prescription, if that makes sense. If a person is having trouble breathing, collecting lots of respiratory oils together means the only result can be their airways open. The same applies for constipation, if you want the loo, you don't want to be messing around with which oil to use. Make a cocktail to give it a right kick up the...

Often when I make a mix, I will make a lot. I'll use a 50ml bottle of carrier and add tons of oils to it. The industry standard for essential oils is that 1 ml = 20 drops (not an exact science because some oils are more viscous than others but it serves a purpose) 50mls then =1000 drops of oil. I can use 1000/25= 40 drops.

Recently I made a blend for a patient with Chronic Pelvic Pain Disorder. I wanted to address the pain and the emotions psychologists suspected might be behind the problem. Actually there are a few drops too many because, in total 43 drops of essential oil found their way in, but that's not enough to worry about. It does mean though, my patient can enjoy the effects of many oils little and often. It's very strong, but far more effective than doing a small mix which could contain fewer oils.

So...

Start off small and add more if you are not seeing the effects you want. If I make it to five drops and cannot see the desired effects, then I feel I probably have picked the wrong oils and blend again. There are rare occasions when I use more, but they are few and far between. You will see, in the blends by other therapists though, sometimes they will lean very heavily on one certain oil. One of the reasons for this is to make it act on more levels. By adding more drops of an oil it raises its vibration and shifts it from physical uses to emotional and spiritual aspects. This is covered more in *Essential Oils for the Mind Body Spirit - The Holistic Medicine of Clinical Aromatherapy* .

Carrier Oils

Without fail your essential oils should be diluted in some sort of carrier. The most common of these are - carrier oils. These are macerations of oils, or sometimes they are cold pressed. Whilst they do not have the potency of an essential oil they do nevertheless have their own properties and can be extremely useful to add to your treatments.

Each oil looks very different and has a different texture and consistency to it too. Calendula is bright sunshine yellow. Tamanu is a slightly unpleasant dark murky green. Sea Buckthorn is a sharp bright orange. You will want to consider this when using for massage, and when you add to a cream or lotion it will change the appearance of that too. We are not quite talking as drastic a mistake as massaging with beetroot juice, but even so there may be staining concerns.

They will not only enhance the properties of your essential oils but carrier oils improve creams and lotions no end. They thicken the structure of the cream and add a luscious silkiness to it. Best of all is how much cheaper they are than essential oils so you can add a brilliant new dimension to a cream without spending much money at all. As a guide for measuring, you probably need about a teaspoon of carrier to each 4 drops of essential oil. There is no need to increase the amount of essential oil by very much just because you add more carrier. Remember it is the essential oils that do the heavy lifting, the carrier is nothing more than the cart to transport them. Mess around with the carrier to get your consistency right and make sure that you have enough oil for each treatment.

A note of caution is the fact many of these oils are cold pressed from nuts. Since it seems nut allergies are on the rise (or at least awareness of them seems to be, anyway) you should consider this each time you make a treatment for someone. Be aware the kernel of a fruit can cause the same reactions as can the seed, so peach kernel, camellia, jojoba, tamanu and apricot kernel should be added to your *use-with- caution* list.

Carrier oils tend to come in between 100-500ml bottles. The temptation might be to buy a larger bottle for economy, but ensure you will use it enough. Carrier oils mostly start to go rancid between 6-12 months because they oxidise pretty quickly.

All that being said, don't feel you have to rush out and buy any of these. The vegetables oils, grapeseed, sunflower, rapeseed or olive oils you have on the shelf to cook with at home are wonderful in their own rights. Olive oil is thicker and so feels delicious for the person receiving the massage, but you will feel you have worked harder at the end of it. Grapeseed is one of the thinnest oils, gives good slip on the skin and helps essential oils to absorb into the skin quickly.

Remember the most important uses of these carrier oils, over and above their properties, are to dilute the essential oils to a dose which your skin can easily handle, to help them absorb through the skin easily and to break them down small enough for your liver and kidneys to be able to assimilate them when it comes to eliminating waste.

There are many carrier oils on the market today, so I have included a short list of some of my favourites with their uses. When you tire of using the sunflower, olive or groundnut oils you have in the cupboard, here are some more you may enjoy experimenting with:

Almond Oil

(Nut*) – This is a fab oil to add to blends that feel too thin. It is a thick robust oil and you only need about a teaspoonful to make the mix thick and luxurious to use. It is very smoothing and plumping to the skin so is delicious to add to face masks too.

Apricot Kernel

(Nut*) – This is a medium consistency oil with a very pale peach-y hue. It would be my choice to treat any problem where there is inflammation. So, perhaps a swollen ankle, or very fiercely red skin might be good examples. It is soothing and reduces inflammation very quickly.

Borage

I would use this for eczema as it has a high gamma linolenic acid content. It is also extremely effective at cleansing the liver (which is also a concern with eczema. See *The Essential Oil Liver Cleanse* and *The Aromatherapy Eczema Treatment*). Borage is a thin and colourless oil.

Calendula

A cheaper alternative to the essential oil this is a very caring skin healer. See details for the essential oil and also the extra article on calendula that shows how to use this oil to help radiation burns after cancer treatments. Of all skin healers, this is my favourite.

Camellia

This thin, colourless oil is cold pressed from the seed. It is bursting with Omega 6. This is a naturally occurring fatty acid that the body uses to regenerate tissues. I love this oil for mature skins because it refines them, softens them and helps the body to bring younger, newer skin cells to the surface. This is an emollient oil, and it helps the skin to retain moisture. Use, then, to thicken moisturisers. This will work best if used in conjunction with regular facial massage to reveal fresher skin cells too.

Use also for hair treatments, nails and cuticles too.

Coconut

(Nut*) – This one is a book in its own right, there are so many uses. Use for very dry and brittle hair to add moisture. Excellent for sports massage because it helps the body to burn energy far more efficiently. I use it mostly for carrying oils when I want an antibacterial kick though. Coconut is antibacterial and antifungal.

Evening Primrose

Ooo this is deliciously thick unguent oil. The bright yellow hue betrays how laden it is with GLA. This component is wonderfully healing to the skin. It is a useful carrier to use in your treatments of eczema and psoriasis but also for gynaecological care too. I would not suggest massage for broken skin conditions such as eczema, not least because it is likely to be embarrassing to the patient, but a cream or lotion with this added can be beautiful.

Hazelnut

(*Nut) One of the nut oils, obviously, it oozes vitamin E so is a fabulous skin food. By far its best action is the way it will exfoliate the skin. Use it as your facial massage and after a moment or two you will feel grittiness under your fingers as the dead skin cells slough off.

Jasmin

Now this is one of my favourite carriers because if you know where to look it can be a delicious bargain. Check out Asian grocery stores and even the Indian aisles in supermarkets. It is a wonderful nourishment for the hair and is used extensively for daily treatments in Ayurvedic medicine. It carries the same properties as jasmine essential oil so use it for preparations where there may be scarring, for gynaecological complaints that may include the need for a uterine tonic. I would avoid using if for oily skins/ acne though, simply because this golden yellow oil is so very thick it is just too heavy for the already greasy complexions.

Jojoba

This oil is cold pressed from the seed. It is a very good skin stabilizer. Treat both oily and dry skins with jojoba because it helps to *balance* sebum production, turning the tap on or off as needed. This is another good carrier to moisturise cuticles. It is especially helpful with false nails because it nourishes the nail beds too, which might otherwise become damaged.

Peach Kernel

(Nut*)– This is the perfect match to go with Neroli essential oil when you are treating more mature skins. It helps to plump the skin and smooth lines. It has high concentrations of vitamins A & E and because it is a very thin and light oil, is better for skins that are prone to blocked pores too.

Rosehip

Again we have a skin regeneration product here. Use on damaged complexions, rosacea and acnes, for instance. I also find it useful after a wound has healed to avoid scarring. This is a gentle oil and so would be my oil of choice for children, rather than jasmine which has a bit too much sass for kids, somehow.

Sea Buckthorn

This is a super-oil. It is on my bucket list to find these growing naturally and squeeze the oil straight from the berry into my hand. Use for any problem where there is congestion, phlegm, catarrh, constipation, even impacted skin...that list is endless. It is a fiercely efficient skin healer, by that I mean it heals quickly, but is not gentle, so avoid on skins that are sore. It has very low skin protection from the sun too, so is useful for moisturisers whilst you are on holiday. (It is not strong enough to replace a sunscreen though.) It is too strong to use as a massage oil on its own and will severely stain the skin. Use not more than a teaspoon in a mix or just a few drops into a cream or lotion.

St John's Wort

This comes from the beautiful yellow flowered bush Hypericum. You may have noticed it has a scarlet bud and this is where the oil comes from. The bright red hue of the oil betrays its source. It is a useful choice for conditions with aches and pains, whether that is rheumatism or arthritis even sports massage. It is also helpful for treating symptoms of stress incontinence. St John's Wort is safe to use but can neutralise the effects of many drugs. When I checked the database today there was 729 contraindicated drugs (5027 brand and generic names) and of course as more drugs come on the market I suspect that number will also grow. In order to keep the safety data as current as I can, I have added link at buildyourownreality.com/resources/

Tamanu

(Nut*) This dark green oil has more clinical than beauty applications. It is anti-inflammatory, anti-neuralgic and is skin healing too. Again, this is too thick and green to be the only oil in your massage treatment, perhaps blend with grapeseed.

Walnut

(Nut*) – The very best walnut oil is Topaz blue, but it is rare to find this. Mostly yours will be fairly translucent, and that quality is fine to use. This is a very good oil to increase circulation and also to boost hormonal levels.

Where to apply essential oils

As explained, oils absorb through the skin, into the blood stream. This means they can get to the spot that needs them wherever your place them onto the skin. Here's a nice experiment for you.

Rub a clove of garlic on the soles of your feet (not on a night of planned romance please!!!), then 20 minutes later garlic can be smelt on your breath. That is because the essential oils have travelled around the body via the blood system.

It makes sense though, that the closer to the site of pain you can get, the more effective your therapy will be. I also find it helpful to apply the oils on two other spots.

Turn your hand palm up and you will notice blue veins in your wrist. This is an excellent blood supply close to the surface and so works very well for fast administration of oils.

For infection issues, coughs, colds etc I also rub down the side of the neck where the lymphatic system drains, just below the collar bone. The lymphatic system has several functions but notably here it combats infection and removes waste cells and products from the system.

Ways to apply essential oils

Creams and lotions

This is a great way of using essential oils because it means you can administer little and often. It is possible to make them, but it is fiddly and quite expensive to do. Jill Bruce sells blank creams and lotions in her store, The Apothecary. You can find a link to her store in the directory (pg 381). These are my preferred way of administering oils. You simply add however many drops you need to use and stir them in.

Massage Oils

I have included a section on massage and of course this would be the preferred method of application for this, but actually massage oils can be used at any time. The vegetable oil is nothing more than a means of diluting the oil to transport it through the skin.

In the bath

Wallow in luxury, and I promise you nothing else really comes close to the relaxation of an aromatherapy bath. I tend not to make bath oils, rather a few drops straight in the water serves just as well. If you do have a contact who is an aromatherapist, ask them to make you a bath oil, because you can benefit from several oils at once rather than paying out for bottle after bottle of more costly essential oils.

Diffusers

These have come a long way over the twenty years since I trained. Then you had to have a little candle under a warm bowl of water for the oils to diffuse. Now there are electronic gadgets to do the trick and they are ace.

Once the oils evaporate they entirely change the atmosphere of the room. This is wonderful for also changing people's moods, you can uplift, soothe arguments or even seduce. On a physical level this is useful for headaches, nausea, insomnia and breathing complaints in particular.

Candles

This is at the very forefront of my mind at the moment as I am designing a range to help with the emotional fall out from terminal illness. They need not be used for anything quite so serious though. Simply choose uplifting oils, relaxing, stimulating or whatever effect you are looking for, to make your candle.

The easiest way is with a sheet of beeswax which you can buy from most craft shops or direct from a beekeeper. (Ebay quite often list them too)

The sheets come in rectangles and you can get 4 candles from each one. Cut the rectangle in half vertically and then cut each section diagonally to create two triangles.

Smear some essential oil down the vertical edge of your triangle. Let it dry for a few moments then take a piece of cotton string to make a wick. Lay it along the same vertical side then crease a small line of the beeswax against the wick to hook it into place.

Roll the beeswax snugly around the wick. Wind it as tightly as you can against the string. Trim the wick to length.

Some people prefer to put the essential oil directly onto the wick but as it burns you lose the freshness of the scent that way.

Room sprays
These are a great way to clean your surroundings. You might want to cleanse the air of bugs hanging about when the kids bring coughs and colds home, or perhaps simply refresh the scent of laundry and linen.

If you don't like using chemical cleaning products, these are good to wipe down surfaces, telephones and light switches where dirt and germs like to breed.

Find yourself an atomiser spray. I use the ones you mist plants with. Use 12 drops of oil to a 50 ml bottle.

Now you can simply add the oils to distilled or tap water, but you will find the oils sink to the bottom. To break down the oils a little I add a teaspoon of vodka into the mix which also prevents oily stains on your lavender scented linen.

Steam Inhalations

Great for colds because it helps to unblock the sinuses, but I also do one of these once a week in my skin care regime to unblock the pores and really let the grime come away.

A small warning that some asthmatics have reported inhalations set off their symptoms. If you do start to cough and wheeze, stop the treatment immediately.

Any size bowl will do for this treatment, but I use my pyrex apple crumble dish because it is big enough to get a good coverage of steam to my face but small enough to make a airtight tent with the towel!

Fill with boiling water, and add about 3 drops of essential oil.

KEEP A GOOD 6 - 8 INS AWAY FROM THE BOWL – any closer and you will scald your face.

Make a tent over your head with the towel so no steam can escape.

How long...?

My record is 2 mins 56 secs....make sure you post in the reviews if you beat it!!! No blowing your nose or wiping your face in the middle, mind!!! Let's see who is made of the hardest stuff!!!!

Compresses

There are two types of compresses, hot and cold. To choose which one to use, think about the effect you want to bring about. Heat will open up and release tissues, cold will cease and tighten them. Any condition where you would have stuck a bag of peas on, use a cold compress, to relax something, use warm.

Hot compress

Fill the washing up bowl with just warmer than hand hot water and then add 5 drops of essential oil. Soak your compress and wring out well. Place on the affected part, and keep warm with a hot water bottle on top. Leave for 5 minutes.

Cold Compress

Same as above with cold water and substitute water bottle for ice or that same bag of peas! Ensure you keep the patient warm because temperature can drop very quickly doing this.

It can be useful to use both. Imagine a rather revolting pus filled ulcer and we want to draw the poison out. Then we would use warm to open the tissues, and cold to close them to rest, then when we open them again with a warm compress, it draws the poison must faster. Alternating compresses makes a suction action which is very efficient.

What is important to remember is when you draw toxins out into a compress, it brings body salts with it. These are very corrosive to towels!! Don't throw your towel in the laundry basket and forget about it because when you come to wash it…it will be full of holes! Wash out compresses immediately. Many people use pieces of muslin, I just use an old towel.

Homeopathic Dose

1/15th of a drop

This is one of my own favourite methods of using essential oils. Sometimes an oil is too harsh (like camphor for instance) or would smell hideous in a blend (you might think cade, I couldn't possibly comment) but I feel I need "the vibration" of the oil. Then I take some carrier oil and count out 14 drops and add one drop of essential oil. I can then use just 1/15 of a drop. It is worth having a diluted bottle in your box or this becomes rather tedious doing it over and over again!

Neat

In France, where the therapists undergo a much more in depth training than anywhere else in the world, aromatherapists sometimes use oils neat on the skin. These are in cases where the therapist has taken a very full case history and is working at a deep level with the patients.

It is best for the untrained therapist to remain within the confines of using diluted essences which are easily strong enough to do their jobs. Many oils cause sensitisation through undiluted use (in particular Tea tree) and can become very painful experiments.

There are a couple of exceptions that prove that rule.

- Use lavender neat on a burn, pour it on with gusto, it will heal it far better than anything else will.

- Dab neat lavender onto teenage spots. It will balance the sebum production and attack any bacteria causing the break out.

- Use lemon and tea tree neat on warts and verrucae. Apply with a cotton bud and avoid the skin surrounding because lemon in particular can burn.

Otherwise, unless instructed by a qualified practitioner, please dilute the oils.

You may come across three alternative methods of application that seem to contradict me here. So I will cover each in turn simply for clarification.

In the States, Australia, and other countries, three methods of application have become popularised that use neat oils as a standard treatment.

Raindrop Technique and Neuro Auricular Technique both pioneered by Dr Gary Young of Young Living Essential oils fame and Aromatouch technique trademarked by doTERRA.

The Raindrop Technique

This method uses 7 single essential oils and 2 essential oil blends placed strategically along the spine, the neck and the feet. The oils are used neat and the treatment lasts around about an hour. The idea of this treatment is very much about balancing and releasing the bodily systems. Some therapists report the method is so relaxing to the spine that their patients are ½ ins taller after the treatment.

Neuro- auricular Technique (NAT)

This technique was first pioneered to help Parkinson's disease patients by an aromatherapist Gary Young. It involves using a rounded probe to massage neat essential oils into the base of the skull and certain vertebrae to connect the physical body and the emotional mind.

Aromatouch

This method of massage involves massaging neat essential oils into energy channels in the body called meridians. You might recognise these as the lines an acupuncturist follows to heal the body.

The Alliance of Aromatherapy recently released the following declaration:

Raindrop technique (RDT), Aromatouch and similar techniques do not meet the criteria for safe practice, as defined by the AIA Standards of Practice. There have been reported adverse effects regarding RDT, in particular. These techniques are typically practice as a one size fits all technique and may not be suitable for people with compromised liver and kidney function, those with heart disease, those on blood thinning medicine, those with allergies to aspirin and other disorders.

alliance-aromatherapists.org

For the purposes of this book, I would like to state I agree with their stance. I do use a very similar way of treating patients to Aromatouch, myself, but use oils that have been diluted.

Essential oils are extremely powerful medicines. I'll take you right back to where you and I came in and remind you…they have <u>*many benefits*</u>. You have no idea of what lurks beneath the skin (I had a blood clot in my lungs that doctors suspect formed five weeks before on a plane journey….the body hides things for a long time before you notice them).

Please do not use essential oils undiluted on the skin, do not take internally, vaginally or rectally, unless prescribed by a qualified practitioner…and even then expect to regret the tea tree on a tampon treatment for thrush within seconds of doing it. Every new aromatherapist has done it…..but only once. If nothing else, your eyes water, and then if you are a complete wuss like me…you start to cry.

Safety data

Essential oils are not suitable for everyone. The way they encourage the hormones in the systems to alter can create damaging effects in some groups.

The main people to have concerns are:

1. Diabetes sufferers
2. Epilepsy patients
3. Pregnant women
4. Breast feeding women

Diabetes

People with diabetes can safely use most essential oils with the exception of angelica oil. It is worth keeping essential oils containing high ketone content to a minimum especially when the diabetes symptoms are erratic. Oils high in ketones are:

- Peppermint - Mentha x piperita
- Rosemary ct camphor - Rosmarinus officinalis ct camphor
- Rosemary ct verbenone - Rosmarinus officinalis ct verbenone/camphor
- Sage (Spanish) - Salvia lavandulifolia
- Spearmint - Mentha spicata

- Spike Lavender - Lavandula latifolia
- Turmeric - Curcuma longa
- Valerian (Root) - Valeriana officinalis
- Vetiver - Vetiveria zizanoides

Dill and fennel however, are balancing to the pancreas and as such these are very helpful to suffers.

Epilepsy

Neuro-toxic oils, dangerous not only to sufferers of epilepsy but also some types of schizophrenia too, are: **Rosemary, fennel, sage, eucalyptus, hyssop, camphor and spike lavender (Lavendula latifolia)** These are best avoided by these sufferers

Pregnant Women

The many actions that essential oils have, make essential oils dangerous in pregnancy. **All essential oils should be avoided during the first 16 weeks**. Throughout the rest of the pregnancy *avoid Angelica, Black Pepper, Clove, Cypress, Eucalyptus, Ginger, Helichrysum, Marjoram, Myrrh, Nutmeg, Oregano, Peppermint, Roman*

Chamomile, Basil, Cassia, Cinnamon bark, Clary Sage, Lemongrass, Rosemary, Thyme, Vetiver, Wintergreen, White Fir.

Breastfeeding women

The taste of essential oils oozes through into breast milk and so you may find it puts baby off feeding. There are some oils however which the breast feeding mum may find useful. Carrot Seed Oil enhances milk flow, geranium soothes engorged breasts and Marigold heals cracked nipples. All others should be used with care.

If baby does stop feeding stop using oils for a day and see what happens.

Massage

Different types of massage

There are many different types of massage. Aromatherapy massage is often offered in beauty salons. The strokes in an aromatherapy massage are long sweeping strokes. The rest of the treatment benefits of course come from the essential oils themselves. For deeper muscle work, seek out a therapist who offers shiatsu and may also implement acupressure points to help the body detoxify its self even deeper.

To alleviate the friction between the skin and the masseur's hands, we use a carrier. In aromatherapy we use vegetable oils but also talcum powder works very well to let the hands slip easily over the skin. This is often used in Swedish massage.

Benefits of Massage

What a world we live in. We have a fantastic playground close to where I live. The children of tourists from all around the world congregate on the steps of the zip slide to have a go. Most of them aren't tall enough to get on, so they need an extra little shove up. In years gone by you would have stuck a hand under their bum and given them a boost. Life's just not like that anymore and so the other parents just have wait slightly uncomfortably until the fed up kid's mum or dad comes to the rescue. Touch of any description is very taboo.

So who do we touch?

Our lovers; deep in the darkness of night? Snogging in broad daylight seems to be OK for the youth. The rest of us look on with slight discomfort and a tinge of envy that those days of gay abandon are behind us.

I suspect anyone who has found their way to this book, is fairly comfortable hugging a child. But there are many children who don't enjoy the security of an innocent bed time cuddle.

Our pets get a fairly good deal on the stroking front, but people not so much nowadays. In many cases a nurse even has to don a protective pair of rubber gloves to protect herself and her patient.

The age of innocence is gone. So touch, from a relative stranger, is quite an extraordinary thing if you think about it. To enjoy a massage you have to submit your trust completely to a person. It is not easy for many people to do.

In some strange way I suppose you could think of it a bit like the dominatrix and her client. He lies there because he no longer wants to be in control, even just for a few moments, he wants to submit. Massage is the non-sexual version of this. Take off your clothes, strip away responsibility for half an hour.

The mind switches off...if you are lucky, but it is not an automatic response. If a person is having a massage for the first time, they may giggle. Vulnerable at lying with no clothes on, and of course it could be the therapist has not judged their hand pressure correctly...and it tickles!

Try to be the opposite of the hair dresser when you are massaging someone. Don't try to engage them in conversation, just let them drift. Occasionally check your hand pressure is not to hard or too light, ensure they are warm enough, and of course let them know if you want them to turn over.

The Physical Effects of Massage

The skin is the largest organ in the body. It is covered in tiny pores which allow essential oils to enter your body and start doing whatever good you require of them. By rubbing the skin, you warm it. One of the skin's functions is to control body temperature so, as it rises, the pores open more. This allows even quicker admission for the oils. The chemicals speedily enter tiny capillaries on the base layer of the skin and flush around the blood system.

Beneath the skin are muscles. There are several different types of muscle which are all constructed in different ways (for example cardiac muscle) but the ones sitting atop your bones are constructed from many bundles of fibres.

When a muscle works it creates a waste product called lactic acid. This should be removed from the body by the lymphatic system. If the muscles have been working harder than normal though, not all the acid is removed. Over time this crystalises and becomes painfully trapped between the fibres of your muscles.

Try rolling your neck, can you feel some crunching? Lactic acid crystals. These crystals disintegrate quite well under finger tip touch and so massage is vital for keeping muscle stiffness at bay.

A good masseur listens to their fingers to feel where knots and tightness appear under them. Even though there is a script to a massage, the skill is in knowing where to take a moment to concentrate on a painful spot.

Massage increases both circulation and lymphatic drainage. The job of the lymphatic system is to rid our bodies of waste but also to increase immunity. The system circulates the body in a similar way to the blood system, except where circulation has a pump (the heart), the lymphatic system does not. It relies on muscle compression to move it around the body. It follows then, if someone is lean and fit their immunity is going to be better, but massage actively improves lymphatic efficiency and therefore immunity too.

Breathing plays a vital part in massage. We all know slowing down our breathing reduces heart rate and we feel calmer. But...

The reason we have inspiration and expiration (breathing in and out) is we expire (breathe out) the gas exchange that happens in the blood. We take in oxygen and breathe out carbon dioxide. As you break down knots, you release toxicity and deep breathing evicts the waste gases from the body.

This is a knack. If you ask someone not to hold their breath in any parts of the massage that hurt...they'll think about their breathing and suddenly not be able to breathe easily.

I find a technique called mirroring helps. I actively match their speed of breathing as I massage, and I breathe very deeply and deliberately. Then, I gradually slow down my breathing. As a rapport builds, the patient relaxes into my rhythm and matches with it. Try it; it is a very helpful technique.

Issues in the Tissues

Those who go on to read others of my books will begin to see how much I love the magic that crackles in your hands under a bottle of essential oil. There are lots of things that work as a catalyst for this to happen. The release of memories is one of them.

Believe it or not, memories not only stay in your head. They go into the organs and they also go into the muscles. In the *Essential Oil Liver Cleanse* I get almost embarrassingly excited by how transplanted organs have had memories and experiences from the donor transported to their new host body.

Athletes will tell you about muscle memory too. They actively use repetition to get their muscles to form memories and so therefore habits. Memories stay lodged in the muscles and even after the mind has moved onto something else, they lie there waiting.

Massage twists the fibres, and digs into them and this can disturb, awaken and unlock these hidden memories. Don't be surprised if the person starts to weep for apparently no reason. The memory may not even unfold so they recognise the scene playing out. Only the emotions may come to the surface to be released. Massage on.

I would love to be able to outline the physiology that leads to this strange aspect of healing…but in some ways it's a bit like the magician sawing his assistant in half. I'm not sure I want to know, because analysing it would take that magical crackle away. Massage releases memories. It just does!

Contraindications of massage

There are times when massage is not the appropriate course of therapy to choose.

Over contagious or infections skin conditions

Over the abdomen whilst in pregnancy

Over the abdomen in the first two or three days of menstruation (discomfort)

In cardio vascular conditions except under strict medical guidance: examples of these are thrombosis, phlebitis, angina pectoris and hypertension

Do not massage on:

Areas of varicose veins

Any strange lumps or bumps

Recent scar tissue or open wounds

Areas of unidentified pain or inflammation (medical advice to be sought first)

Any condition being treated by a medical doctor unless he agrees

Do not massage over the spine.

Massage Strokes

There are five basic massage strokes

- Effleurage
- Petrissage
- Friction
- Vibration
- Tapotment

Effleurage are long, languid smoothing strokes. They either go deep into the muscles or superficially slide across the surface of the skin. Always perform them with slow precision in the direction of the heart. These encourage lymph flow. This sedative stroke also physiologically improves the functioning of the muscles by encouraging them to take in more nutrients from the blood.

My favourite effleurage stroke is done by standing at the head of the patient, facing their feet. Turn your hands down to face the floor. Touch finger tips and elbows out.

Place your hands either side of the patient's spine. Push down into the body and then push the flesh away from you down to the hips.

Maintaining pressure swivel the hands to circle under the hips and pull the hands back towards you, up the side of the body to the head.

This effleurage motion is deep pressure. It is very relaxing and extremely efficient.

If you can stand up to do the massage (on a couch) let your body do the work. Step forward then step back onto a bent leg so the full force of your body moves the muscle.

Petrissage rolls or kneads the muscles. Twisting and squeezing the muscle fibres stimulates deep blood flow and it also strengthens the muscle.

Friction strokes are circular movements of the hands. They have a very penetrating action which breaks down very deep knots.

You'll come across a great one of these in the back massage. Lay your hands next to each other, and opposite, so your finger tips lie next to the heel of your other hand. Elbows out. Lay your hands on the same side of the spine, on the back, and sharply pull your elbows into your side causing your hands to swivel outwards moving the flesh quickly with them.

We only use the forearm, hands and fingers to exert pressure onto a limb though **Vibration**. This rapid movement helps to stimulate the nervous system.

Again in the back massage: Place the forearms across the width of the back and very quickly rub back and forth.

Tapotment are the aggressive movements everyone recognises in sports massage. Using a cupped or open hand, the therapist makes a chopping, hacking, beating or cupping action. These strokes stimulate the muscles and dependant on how long it is done for, may sedate or invigorate the tissues. (Short action wakes them up, repeating for several rotations is very sedative)

Hand positioning

One of the many reasons I write about therapy more than I see clients is massage hurts my hands. It is extremely rigorous and so you must ensure you correctly position your hands. Whenever you want to exert pressure, use one hand on top of another and try to lean your weight into it rather than just pushing your hands into the muscle.

When doing little circles with your fingers, lay the fingers of the other had over the top for extra strength.

When using a pincer motion, as you would for massaging the shoulder mantle for example, use the strongest muscles of your hand. To do this put your index finger and thumb at right angles and wiggle your thumb. Where the flap of skin is at the join…that's what you want to aim to be "pinching with". Try it, it's much easier to do than describe!

Always be aware of your back too. Keep it straight or by the time you get half way through you will feel like you need a massage too.

Protection

I have deliberately veered away from talking about the aura and chakras in this book, because they sit more happily in the next book about the mind body and spirit. Ignoring it at this point, however, would be cavalier.

The aura is an energy field around your body. It is like a rainbow emanating around 18 inches from your body. We all have it, even if you are not aware of it. Given the right environment, it can be a magnet for germs and emotional disturbances. You must protect it not only from colds and flu, but also emotional trauma too. (Believe me, or believe me not…ignore this bit at your peril. It won't be long until you are laid up feeling ill because you have caught a bug.) Before every treatment visualise yourself getting into a bubble and surrounding it with light. Let the light go entirely around your aura six times. I also imagine it zipping up like a banana skin around me.

I cannot stress how important this is. You need a separation from your patient. From their emotional drains but also their colds, bugs whatever.

At the end of the treatment I imagine raindrops and washing the psychic gunk away. Again, you will feel so much better if you get into the habit each time you treat someone.

Back Massage

Begin your back massage standing at the head of your patient.

Put your hands either side of the spine, finger tips pointing at each other and do a long sweeping effleurage down the length of their spine, out across the lower back and up the sides of the body. Really push the muscle along and down and then pull it hard towards you.

Do this stroke three long, slow times

Move to the side of the couch and reach right over to the other side of the body with both hands.

Slowly and deliberately pull one hand up and then the other and walk then down to the hips. You are deeply stroking the muscles which surround the ribs.

Go up and down the body 3 times

Keep your hand on the patient, walk up to the head and over to the other side of the couch.

Repeat 3 times.

Now do sets of three tapotment up and down the muscles either side of the spine. Cover them thoroughly.

First cup the hands to be like half a coconut and pummel up and down the spine three times. This is called cupping.

Then, using the sides of your hands, chop like they are knives. This is called hacking.

Now put both your hands twisted on the patients back. The hands are immediately next to one another with fingers pointing at the other arms elbow (imagine 5th position in ballet but with your hands) Press down hard and then let your hands twist away from each other so they exert a twisting mechanism on the muscles. We call this twisting or friction.

Now we want to massage the muscles surrounding the actual shoulder blade. First gently smooth in deep clockwise circles over the massage.

Do a series of tiny circles where basically your fingers are probing for knots and breaking them down.

Now we are going to lift the shoulder bone to get under it. You must do this with confidence!

Put one hand under the patients elbow and take their hand with the other. Gently fold their arm back and up, so the hand is lying on their back, near to their neck and spine, the elbow should be at right angles to the body.

Keep a hold of the elbow and with the side of the other hand "saw" under the scapula gently.

Periodically break off and make your hand into a rigid spider and drum the surface of the scapula with the spider to encourage blood flow. Gently, stroke an effleurage over the muscle to smooth it down. We call this Petrissage.

Do this cycle three times.

Go to the head, retain contact and then do the other shoulder blade.

Come up to the head again and so some gentle work massaging the shoulder mantle. These muscles will be tight and sore so work gently at this point as we return to them later as we work down the front of the body.

Finish the back with 3 very long slow effleurages.

Facial Massage

There are many benefits of facial massage treatments:

- Exfoliate the skin, sloughing off old cells and revealing youthful new cells below

- Relaxation of the muscles

- Stimulation of decongestant pressure points to empty sinus congestion and soothe stress

- It moves sluggish lymphatic fluid, draining away puffiness from the face.

- It feels incredible!

First let's look at what a Facial Massage involves. By no means, is it an exact science. Don't feel you have to follow the book, just get a gist of the motions and then go with the flow. It helps to remember to do each step three times. This will mean the cells get worked well and blood flow will be well stimulated too.

There are three main parts. The first is working the muscles. The second is releasing pressure and the third is moving fluid beneath the skin.

What you must do is always work in circular motions in a flowing manner. This will help to release the dead skin cells.

Start at the centre of the forehead right at the hairline. Using the index fingers in both hands exert fingertip pressure and begin tracing tiny circles in a line out towards the ears.

Line under line keep drawing your circles, gradually working right across and down the forehead until you reach the eyebrows.

Then smooth out the forehead using the thumbs.

Then work along the eyebrows and you may feel some spots which feel very sore. These are acupressure point. Hold the pressure on them until they empty. When you have worked along the top of the brows, repeat underneath them.

Next move down to just under the cheek bones and you will find you can hook your finger under. Work along again and empty any sore points out. As you move along the cheekbones you will arrive at the temples, beside the eyes. Using very light finger tip pressure, gently circle these, which is very relaxing.

Now let's move down the chin. Using your thumb, really work the chin will, releasing muscles but also working the oils deep into the cells. Then work along the jaw towards the ears.

Use your thumb and forefinger in a gentle pinch to squash the tension out of the cells. You may find the outer part of your jaw to be very tender as we tend to store anger and frustration here (grit your teeth?) so work gently, softly and thoroughly.

If you can manage to massage your own neck I would always recommend to do so. Be aware not to rub across the spine, instead focus on releasing the tension in the muscles which sit either side and on your shoulders.

For a moment, just look at your hand. You see the fleshy part between the thumb and forefinger? Use that muscle to pinch into your shoulders you find it far more effective than hurting your fingers!

Under the eyes can become puffy and saggy due to a build up of lymphatic fluid beneath the skin. Using your two index fingers next to each other we will move the fluid on one eye and then the other. Lie your fingers next to each other and gradually push the fluid across toward the ears, down the side of the face, down the side of the neck and then into the collar bone. Your action will be a bit like a tiny "one potato, two potato" game down the face.

Fluid of this nature drains back into the body at this point in the collar bone which we call the subclavian.

Now move to the ears and from the top, gently pinch down the side of the fleshy part. Did you know no-one is born with curled up ears? They bunch up through tension so gently try to unroll them to release the tension.

Be mindful though the ears hold all the same reflex points as the feet do (reflexology) so be careful not to over stimulate any by working them too much.

Lastly now use the flat of your hand to do long fluid relaxing strokes across the entire face. Work upwards so as not to drag the skin down.

In total this would take 20 minutes in a clinical setting.

Try it at home, but for the very best effects, why not see if one of our contributors is in your area and treat yourself to a visit?

Chapter 5 How to blend essential oils

There are many ways to blend oils, some people blend by properties, others by chemical and botanical families. The blends which have the most powerful effects are achieved through *synergistic blending.*

Those for whom this a new term, this is choosing oils which come from one of three groups according to their volatility which in turn affects how fast they evaporate. We say **top**, **middle**, and **base** notes. You might also see the top note referred to as the head note, and the middle called the heart note. These more romantic sounding terms are particularly used in perfumery. When you get the ratios right between the notes you have a great harmony which increases healing further.

This works so well because like everything in the universe, essential oils have a vibration, a wavelength. Light is the highest of the frequencies, sound is lower (hence why we see lightning and thunder trails behind). Einstein discovered there are certain harmonies that are more attractive than others, particularly in music but in all natural laws. If any of you have musical ears, you will know the chord A-C-E is very pleasing to the ear, because they have intervals of a third between them. On a piano if you press two keys next to each other down, the effect is jarring and unpleasant.

Whilst it is harder to articulate in scent than in sound, there are certain oils which smell dreadful together because their vibration is too close.

So...we choose a balance of oils of top, middle and base. This gives us a more rounded fragrance, which is easier to relax into. It also gives the brain more of a chance to read and interpret the oils because they evaporate at different speeds. First the mind encounters the bright, light top notes, then the middle and the earth base notes are the last to evaporate. You may already be familiar with this "dry down" effect when you try on perfume. It takes a while for the fragrance to settle and open out. This is the different notes taking their time.

I am lucky enough to have a strange anomaly called synaesthesia. It used to be thought to happen to around one in 2000 people, now scientists suspect as many as ten times as many people have it. I wonder then, do you?

Synaesthesia is when two senses work involuntarily together. A common example is people see colours when they hear music, the Russian artist Wassily Kandinsky creates beautiful works from listening to music. He paints the colours he hears. David Hockney is believed to have done the same. Some people report of seeing the colour red when they hear a trumpet for instance.

In the same way they might have particular taste or smell linked to another sense.

Nothing quite so peculiar happens to me but I can very clearly hear essential oils. Harmony and discord resound loudly to me in a blend. I try, then, to aim for Mozart over Shostakovich!!!

If you would like a nice representation of this, have a listen to The Heavens are Telling from Hayden's Creation. I have added a link for you on buildyourownreality.com/resources

This will help you to get a feel of how the oils dance in a good blend. Imagine the light citrus sopranos and flutes on the top, kept into check by the myrrh and galbanum basses, and then you have the alto lavender and palma rosa keeping the whole thing in balance.

If the soprano citruses had been the whole blend it would be shrill and sharp, but the middle and base notes anchor it giving it a richness.

There are counterpoint balances where some do more work, and the other parts simply support. Then at the end see how the blend is carefully melded to a crescendo...this is how a really great synergistic blend should work.

I once put this into practice with the Wolverhampton Civic Choir by creating a blend of the notes and putting them into candles for a concert of The Creation. The candles were put into floral arrangements around the church for the performance. The effect was angelic for the audience and choir.

I have attached a separate list of oils and their blending notes, because I like to have mine pinned to the wall for quick reference. You can download the list at buildyourownreality.com/blending-notes

Chapter 6 The List of Ailments

If you take in nothing else from this book, please take this. Alternative medicine is full of people telling you their healing techniques are better than the doctor's. This may or not be true, but these people can be dangerous. Whatever happens, the doctor's advice trumps anything you find in a book like this.

I have been an aromatherapist for 21 years, but I trained for one and then took another year's post grad training. There is no possible way my training can compare to that of an MD or GP. For this reason, I call the medicine I practice Complementary Medicine. It is complementary, in addition, to what the doctor tells you. If you feel more comfortable using my methods, wonderful. Take this book to your physician next time you go. Never, ever give up your medicine, just because an alternative physician told you so.

In some ways aromatherapy and essential oil therapy are different things. At the beginning of the book I referred to holistic approach. In aromatherapy we look at the entire life situation that may have led to the symptoms we see presenting. What follows is list of essential oils that help complaints; reduce the symptoms if you like.

This is not dissimilar to the pill or cream the doctor will give you. The oils are nothing more than salves to ease the symptom for the moment. True aromatherapy looks beneath the surface and asks "But what happened to cause this symptom in the first place?" If you find that as fascinating as I do, then you will enjoy the later books in this Secret Healer series. They open illness cupboards left dusty for many generations and look to see where the disease initially grew from.

Here though are the oils I use to kiss injuries better. Below is simply a list of the oils I would use. Refer to the How to Use Section to find the most suitable way for you to do this for each presenting symptom. You might find it useful to keep a large pot of blank lotion in your fridge to simply use as a carrier each time you want to make up a cream. That way if you only want to make 10ml of a calendula cream for nappy rash, or a small treatment for a hayfever outbreak you can.

Remember in each case, less is more. So even though I have not written amounts, use one or two drops of oil, at the most three. Don't forget too, there is a chart to help you with blending, if you have not yet downloaded it.

Abscess – Galbanum

Aching muscles – Lavender, chamomile, geranium

Acne – Use tea tree to reduce the bacterial infection and jasmine to reduce scarring.

Allergies – Melissa is antihistamine, but for in depth therapy read *The Essential Oil Liver Cleanse* and also *The Aromatherapy Eczema Treatment*

Alopecia – Reputed to be lavender and rosemary massaged into the scalp. Also try argan oil but I have no experience to draw on here

Aphrodisiac -Ylang ylang, sandalwood, rose

You might also like to see the blend done by specialist sex therapist Annie Day (Pg 331).

Appetite – To stimulate appetite - tarragon

Arthritis – Lavender for the pain, Juniper to disperse the uric acid build up

Athletes foot – Tea Tree, use neat and also wash socks with it to kill any lurking microbes

Babies

    Bed wetting – cypress

- **Bruises** – Geranium, use with witch hazel from the chemist and arnica gel.

- **Coughs colds and sneezes** – myrtle.

- **Nightmares/terrors:** lavender, geranium, chamomile and valerian, but I would suggest getting Rock Rose Bach Flower essence

- **Oils to calm frustrated babies** – Lavender, chamomile, geranium, myrtle.

- **Oral thrush** – Tea tree massaged onto the cheeks

- **Problems sleeping** – Lavender, chamomile, catnip, violet leaf, valerian

- **Teething** – Roman chamomile, but homeopathic chamomilla granules from the chemist are probably more effective in my opinion.

- **Tummy upsets** – Dill, spearmint, Chamomile, or mandarin in a lotion or compress.

- **Nappy Rash** – Calendula with a drop of Chamomile maroc blended into a moisturiser, (or I blend into a tub of zinc and castor oil cream)

See also lovely blend for children's cuts and grazes by professional aromatherapist Sharon Falsetto (P343).

Black heads- Grapefruit

Bladder infections – Tea tree, bergamot, cypress, lemon

Blood pressure – ylang ylang balances. Also use geranium to soothe the underlying stress

Breasts, sore – geranium, use warm compresses

Broken skin – Myrrh

Bronchitis – Eucalyptus, Inula, myrrh, bergamot, tea tree

Bruising – geranium also use arnica and witch hazel (herbals not essential oils)

Burns – Neat lavender

Candida – Geranium, lemon for full therapy see *Aromatherapy Eczema Treatment*

Cellulite – Grapefruit, fennel, juniper, cypress

Chicken Pox - again is a herpes virus, but this time herpes zoster. The same applies for shingles. Use mandarin and tea tree in a lotion with lavender and chamomile to sooth the itching.

Circulation – geranium, black pepper

Cold sores – Tea tree neat

Colds Tea tree, Kanuka, Inula, lemon, eucalyptus

Colic – Dill, use in lotion or compress

Colitis – coriander, cardamom, Chamomile

Concentration – frankincense, rosewood, melissa

Constipation – ginger, black pepper, cardamom, coriander, dill, Chamomile

Cough – myrtle, inula

Cystitis – tea tree, bergamot

Depression- This is covered in much more depth in Essential oils for the *Essential Oils for the Mind Body Spirit - The Holistic Medicine of Clinical Aromatherapy* . See Emotions. Also see the blend for depression by Dave from Cambridge Aromatherapy (pg 335).

Dermatitis – Calendula (see The Aromatherapy Eczema Treatment)

Diarrhoea – Tea tree, dill, ginger, cypress

Dry skin – Rose, geranium, frankincense

Eczema – Geranium, Calendula (See The Aromatherapy Eczema Treatment)

Emotions – Covered in depth the Essential Oils for the *Essential Oils for the Mind Body Spirit - The Holistic Medicine of Clinical Aromatherapy*. Meanwhile I have included a small chart to keep you going, published by kind permission of The Garden of Eden and Jill Bruce, from where much of the information came. Download it at buildyourownreality.com/oils-for-emotions

Fever – Camphor (Homeopathic dose only and not on children). For children use 1 drop peppermint on a cold flannel.

Fibromyalgia – Yarrow, spikenard, rosemary, chamomile matricaria.

Flatulence – dill, carrot seed.

Gingivitis - lemon

Gout - juniper

Haemorrhoids – geranium in a cold compress or cream

Halitosis – dill, peppermint

Headaches – lavender. Rosemary for nerve pain

For in depth therapy see the Essential Oil Migraine Treatment

Herpes

The herpes simplex is responsible for a large number of conditions including chicken pox, shingles and cold sores. This is a virus we all carry around with us naturally. It throws up other illnesses when we catch an infection of some description, hence the name cold sores, (we get them when we have a cold.)

Tea tree is a wonderfully anti viral oil and I would suggest using neat onto the cold sore blister. Ensure you wash your hands before and after.

Genital herpes is also thrown up by the same simplex and so still use tea tree, but I would also use bergamot since it has such a wonderful affinity with the genito- urinary system.

A wash of these oils is very useful here but it does need to be very weak, otherwise it will really sting. Dilute 5 drops of tea tree and bergamot in a table spoon of vodka then add to 250 ml of cool boiled water. Keep in a dark bottle and wash using it twice a day.

You might also want to visit the blend for shingles Jill Bruce.

Hyperactivity

Lavender, Chamomile, geranium, frankincense, valerian, rosewood

A 2011 study of hyperactivity in attention Deficit Disorder in Egyptian Children showed the children all had significant deficits in Magnesium, Zinc and a protein that carries iron around the body called ferritin.

I am a massive advocate of magnesium and in *The Essential Oil Liver Cleanse* I show evidence of just how many people are magnesium deficient, and how this is thought to be leading to Non Alcoholic Fatty Liver Disease contributing to everything from eczema and allergies to heart disease and strokes.

I would begin by saying no matter which oils you choose, make magnesium and zinc supplements your first port of call. Vitamin therapy and emotional responses are covered in more depth in *The Professional Stress Solution* but:

For oils see the emotions chart at buildyourownreality.com/oils-for-the-emotions

IBS

The best results I have seen have been to take Aloe Vera juice orally.

Essential oils- *Neroli, cardamom, coriander, Chamomile maroc, carrot seed and dill.*

This is an illness which is completely rooted in emotional disturbance so to conquer this you will need also to read on to Essential Oils of the *Essential Oils for the Mind Body Spirit - The Holistic Medicine of Clinical Aromatherapy* .

Impotence

Nutmeg oil. Also use aphrodisiac oils. For more focused therapy read *The Professional Stress Solution* to understand why this may be happening and treat the underlying cause.

Infection –Tea tree, Manuka, Kanuka, Cinnamon leaf, thyme

Insomnia- Lavender and chamomile to soothe. Marjoram works on the central nervous system to help the body clock. Also treat the probable stress cause.

Neuralgia or nerve pain – Rosemary - not suitable for sufferers of epilepsy.

Oily Skin – Lavender which will balance sebum production.

Open pores – Myrtle

Pregnancy, Labour – See safety on Pg 14 and massage oil and bath oil labour blends by Midwife Sue Mousley on Pg 349.

Psoriasis – Cajuput, Bergamot, lavender, chamomile

Relaxation – Lavender, Chamomile, Ylang ylang, geranium, sandalwood, bergamot, myrrh, valerian...there are too many to mention. For really deep relaxation, why not try some hypnotherapy too? There is a free download (Normally retails at £9.99, free with this book) generously given by Mark Bowden Hypnotherapy available at buildyourownreality.com/ free-hypnosis-download

Rheumatism – Lavender for the pain, juniper for uric acid

Shingles - See blend by Jill Bruce of The Apothecary Pg 347

Sinusitis – Myrrh, lemon, frankincense, eucalyptus, inula. See the section on how to give a facial massage. Focus on the sinus acupressure points. For deeper therapy see the *Essential oils sinus treatment*

Sore throats – One drop each of tea tree and lavender in a pint of water. Gargle it to help the pain and to wash away bacteria. Because I am a wuss who always has man-flu...I add an aspirin to the water too!!!

Sports injuries:

- **Aching joints** – lavender eases the pain and juniper flushes out the lactic acid build up. Perfect in the bath after the first exercise session after a long break.

- **Ballerina Toes** – Use myrrh or galbanum to heal where pointe shoes rub.

- **Broken bones** – more herbal than aromatherapy, but comfrey either used as leaves under a bandage, a maceration or contact a herbalist.

- **Bruises** – Geranium, use with witch hazel from the chemist and also arnica gel. See also recipe by Natalie Miller on Pg 364.

- **Muscle strain** lavender, juniper, black pepper, geranium

- **Sprained ankle** – Lavender for discomfort, geranium and fennel to flush out the swelling, frankincense for the connective tissue.

- **Tendons** – Frankincense brings back elasticity, lavender eases the pain

Spots – Lavender oil or tea tree oil neat on the spot. If spots are a recurring problem add cypress, grapefruit and bergamot to your skin care creams

Stretch marks – Coconut oil. Rub gently into your belly.

Thrush – Tea tree and bergamot. See also candida

Toothache – Your grandma was right. Sorry despite the revolting taste...clove oil. Use lavender, spikenard or yarrow for really acute pain.

Varicose veins – Geranium oil in a lotion. No massage, only gently stroke in the lotion.

Verruca- Take a cotton bud and put lemon oil and tea tree neat onto the verruca. Do not touch the surrounding skin as it will cause skin sensitization

Warts – see verruca

Wrinkles – Neroli and camellia carrier, as well as frankincense.

Worms - Thyme

Chapter 7 Choosing Essential Oils

How to build an essential oils collection

The first questions someone always asks me are what are the best oils to get. This is very much subjective, based on how much you will use them, but, to my mind....

The most useful oils to have in your box are

- Lavender
- Chamomile
- Geranium
- Tea Tree
- Myrrh
- Rose
- Cinnamon
- Marigold
- Sandalwood
- Frankincense

Closely followed by

- Grapefruit
- Cedarwood (Atlas)
- Cypress
- Ylang Ylang
- Rosemary
- Jasmine
- Valerian
- Eucalyptus
- Inula

I am sure though, as you make your way through the hundred or so oils profiles, there will be some that speak to you more than others. With my bad lung, for instance, I have an enviable stash of respiratory oils. A person with IBS is more likely to have hoarded digestive oils.

I have included the phrase:

Historical successes of using this **essential oil** have included:

into each section which should give you an indication of **how it has been extracted.** Where appropriate I have added the methods of extraction for you so you will have essential oil by steam or hydro distillation and absolutes by enfleurage, solvent or CO_2 extraction. Producers however, experiment with extractions and so there may be more products available than the list. By its very nature, it cannot be all encompassing. Some producers for example offer lavender oil absolutes, and *Rose maroc* might be extracted by enfleurage or *Rose otto* by distillation. Whilst the properties of the plant may remain similar, clearly the chemical composition may change with a differing method of extraction and so you might find it to be "more analgesic", "more astringent" etc. etc.

The main list is a first aid check list, really. Consider these to be band aids when you need them most. After that I have included some bonus material of a new product I shall be launching in 2015 of profiles of single essential oils. There are 6 of these and more will go on sale next year should you want to add them to your reference files. Consider them to be "Everything you ever wanted to know about lavender, chamomile, tea tree, rose, myrrh and geranium".

The in depth profiles show how clinical trials are working towards licensed drugs made from active components of our plant medicines. Use the information contained in them how you will. Clearly, because a rat has recovered from diabetes because he has been treated with a certain oil does that mean a person certainly will. But a professional aromatherapist might consider that it *may* and think about including it in their next diabetic patient's blend. This experimentation is what moves our industry forward. The rodent trials are early indicators of a plant's usefulness, but before a drug is released it must undergo many more studies including those on human volunteers, not only to test efficacy, but also safety. So then, in some ways, at this moment in time, our primitive medicine could be considered to be often ahead of its time. It is a fascinating time for plant healing.

You will also find links to articles as you go through too. Over the years I have written many millions of words about aromatherapy on different websites. Many of these are on oils and absolutes which are not really covered in other books because they are less well known choices. Amazon restricts the amount of content I can duplicate in this book and on websites to just 10%. Rather than playing around and altering old stuff, I have placed some of these more interesting articles in pdfs for you to download and place into your references too. There are articles attached to Catnip, Damiana, Agarwood, Calendula as well as articles I have published in professional aromatherapy journals on Galbanum and Tuberose. Please do take advantage of these. They are fairly big files that will add a great deal over and above what you find in this book.

Notes about regulation and legislation

Whilst there is no over arching regulatory body of aromatherapy, we do have membership organisations who promote good practice in our industry. We are also controlled by a degree by the FDA (America) and the Medicines Control's Board (UK). These organisations protect the general public by restricting what we can and can't say aromatherapy can do because they have not yet undergone these tests and come out the other side successfully.

Firstly: As an aromatherapist, I can't say we can **cure** *anything, merely that essential oils may optimise, maintain or support certain functions.*

Because oils have not yet undergone rigorous testing to see if an oil will successfully perform in the same manner each time it is used, (costing thousands upon thousands of pounds) we must also be very careful we do not suggest an essential oil might be a drug to treat a condition. In practical terms this means, if I made you a pot of cream for your eczema, whilst you would call it your eczema cream, I would have to label it as lavender, Chamomile and geranium or whichever oils I decided to put in.

So...

Please note, the below is not designed to be a list of cures, however historically these oils have been used on patients with these conditions and have seen positive outcomes. If you were to approach a qualified professional aromatherapist, these are some of the oils he/she might choose after seeing you for a full face to face consultation.

Should you find there is the odd medical term you do not understand please refer to the medical glossary on Pg 410.

You will notice sometimes an oil might be contra-indicated for certain conditions – for clarity this means do *not* use.

What I must also reiterate here again is: the doctor knows best.

Please, please, please...

Do not abandon your medicines because of anything you have read in this book. By all means take it along to discuss alternatives with the doctor, but his/her word goes.

Lastly: a note a pregnancy. Essential oils should not be used in the first 16 weeks of pregnancy, in my opinion. I have marked some oils as safe to use, but not until after these first four months have elapsed.

That first trimester is such a delicate time, and we cannot predict fully what the effects of an oil are going to be on a growing foetus. In some ways, it could be they are safer, paradoxically, because they do not have the enzymes in their systems to convert some of the chemical reactions that might cause in the liver and kidneys damage in an adult body, for instance. But, likewise there are oils that will cause heavy bleeding, are abortificaent, and can cause immune responses that could be responsible for evicting the embryo. The forming baby is far too precious to take the risk. So for morning sickness, have ginger biscuits and peppermint cordial...lay off the oils please.

The Essential Oils of the Physical Body

Agarwood

Aquilaria malaccensis

Historical successes of using this **essential oil** have included:

- Aphrodisiac uses
- Sedative uses
- Anti-inflammatory uses
- Nausea
- Regurgitation
- Smallpox
- Rheumatism
- Illness during and after childbirth
- Relieves spasms of the digestive system and even certain kinds of cancer
- Colic
- Abdominal pain

- Cirrhosis of the liver

- Respiratory systems

- Shortness of breath

- Chills

- General pains

- Asthma

- Weakness in the elderly

- Problems of the urinary tract

- Relieves epilepsy

- Agarwood Essential Oil works as a director or focuser for other medicines.

Safety: General regarded as safe.

Agarwood or Oudh is an oil that often gets overlooked, not least because of its massive price tag. I wrote about it in 2009. If you would like to read more in depth information about how it works not only on the physical body, but also for emotional and spiritual aspects, as well as sexuality, feel free to download the article at **buildyourownreality.com/agarwood**

Angelica Root
Angelica archangelica

Historical successes of using this **essential oil** have included:

- Reduction of congestion and calming spasm
- Digestive
- Cramps
- Coughs- asthma, bronchitis, headaches
- Clears phlegm
- Stomach cramps and stomach aches
- Compacted skin or sluggish circulation
- Aids peristalsis and drives gases downwards and out of the body
- Cleanses the blood of toxins and is diuretic
- Rheumatism, arthritis and gout – because it clears uric acid
- Renal tonic – as it clears excess salts

- Promotes sweating – so useful for cleansing toxicity but also reducing fever

- High blood pressure

- Eases the flow of menstruation, makes it more regular and reduces clotting

- Steadies the nerves

- Stimulant to hormones

- Tonic to metabolism and digestion

Safety: General regarded as safe.

Because of high levels of bergamptene, angelica root can be phototoxic. Angelica seed has no such connotations and can be used safely by most, but do not use in pregnancy. Best to be used in dilutions of less than 0.8%. It should not be used by suffers of diabetes. Angelica seed is a far cheaper oil than root and may sometimes be used to cut the more expensive oil.

Anise, Star
llicium verum

Historical successes of using this **essential oil** have included:

- Digestion
- Aches and pains
- Rheumatism
- Colic
- Colds and flu

Hazards: Potentially carcinogenic, based on estragole and safrole content; reproductive hormone modulation; may inhibit blood clotting. Contraindications (all routes): Pregnancy, breastfeeding, endometriosis , estrogen-dependent cancers, children under five years of age.

Anise
Pimpinella anisum

Historical successes of using this **essential oil** have included:

- Nervous dyspepsia
- Flatulence

- Nervous vomiting

- Nauseous migraine

- Vertigo

- Painful periods

- Colic

- Palpitations

- Cough

- Bronchial spasm

Hazards: Potentially carcinogenic, based on estragole content; reproductive hormone modulation; may inhibit blood clotting. Contraindications (all routes): Pregnancy, breastfeeding, endometriosis , estrogen-dependent cancers, children under five years of age.

Basil, sweet

Ocimum basilicum

Historical successes of using this **essential oil** have included:

- Chest infections
- Bronchitis
- Whooping cough
- Reduces fever
- Engorged and painful breasts
- Scant periods
- Digestive problems (gentle abdominal massage)
- Jaundice
- Headaches in particular migraine
- Head colds
- Clears the mind, is cephalic
- Nervous debility,
- Mental fatigue

- Anxiety

- Nervous insomnia

- Gout

- Overall tonic

Safety: Moderate skin irritant, so I would avoid adding to the bath. Not safe for use in pregnancy.

Basil, holy

Ocimum tenuiflorum, you might also see this referred to by its local name Tulsi

Historical successes of using this **essential oil** have included:

- Beautifully sedative and very helpful in easing congestion

- Reduces anything compacted so catarrh, mucous, sinus headaches

- Protects from infection

- Reduces fever

- Boosts immunity

- Lung problems, infections and pain
- Soothes eye infections – styes, conjunctivitis etc
- Soothes the nerves
- Lowers blood pressure
- Protects the teeth and tightens gums
- Ayurveda says retains youth and is anti-aging

Hazards: May contain methyleugenol; drug interaction; may inhibit blood clotting; skin sensitization (moderate risk); mucous membrane irritation (low risk). Cautions: Anticoagulant medication, major surgery, peptic ulcer, haemophilia, other bleeding disorders. Do not use in dilutions of higher than 1%

Bay

Pimenta racemosa

Historical successes of using this **essential oil** have included:

- Digestive
- Eases nerve pains, neuralgia

- Tonic to the liver and kidneys
- Treating strains and sprains
- Dental infections
- Stimulates the scalp so may help hair growth
- Blood thinning

Hazards: Drug interaction; may contain estragole and methyleugenol; may inhibit blood clotting; skin sensitization (low risk); mucous membrane irritation (low risk). Cautions: Anticoagulant medication, major surgery, peptic ulcer, hemophilia, other bleeding disorders. Use in a maximum dilution of 1.8%

Benzoin

Styrax benzoin

Historical successes of using this **absolute** have included:

- Coughs & Colds
- Sore throats
- Constipation

- Mucous complaints
- Helps the flow of urine
- Urinary tract infections
- Excellent skin healer
- Cracked toes, especially dancers pointe shoes

Hazards: Skin sensitization (low risk).

Cautions (dermal): Hypersensitive, diseased or damaged skin, children under 2 years of age.

Bergamot
Citrus bergamia

Historical successes of using this **essential oil** have included:

- Urinary tract infections
- Depression- extremely uplifting
- Anorexia (according to Valnet)
- Regulates appetite

- Dyspepsia

- Intestinal parasites

- Skin infections

- Reduces the effects of the herpes simplex (cold sores, chicken pox, shingles etc)

- Keeps dogs and cats off the grass!!!!

Safety: General regarded as safe.

Hazards: Phototoxic (moderate risk); may be photocarcinogenic. Contraindications (dermal): If applied to the skin at over maximum use level, skin must not be exposed to sunlight or sunbed rays for 12 hours. Cautions: Old or oxidized oils should be avoided. Maximum dermal use level: 0.4% to avoid phototoxicity.

Bergamot FCF presents none of the above hazards

Birch, white
Betula alba

Historical successes of using this **essential oil** have included:

- Muscular aches and pains

- Severe eczema and psoriasis (there are gentler options)

- Clears and opening the respiratory tract

Safety: Moderate risk of skin irritation. Do not use in pregnancy.

Black Pepper

Piper nigrum

Historical successes of using this **essential oil** have included:

- Digestive

- Warming

- Antispasmodic (to the gut)

- Stimulates the kidneys

- Anaemia, stimulates the spleen

- Muscular pain and fatigue

Safety: Moderate risk of skin irritation, so do not use in the bath. Do not use in pregnancy.

Bois de Rose

See rosewood

Cade

Juniperus oxycedrus

Historical successes of using this **essential oil** have included:

- Eczema, dermatitis, psoriasis and skin problems
- Herpes syntax – cold sores, chicken pox
- Alopecia
- Allergic rhinitis
- Stuffy nose

Safety: Do not use in pregnancy. Always look for labelling of rectified on cade oil. It is a very potent oil, unrectified cade oil is be carcinogenic. This oil is however best avoided.

Cajuput

Melaleuca cajeputi

Historical successes of using this **essential oil** have included:

- Inhalations and colds
- Inhibits bacteria
- Sore throats, headaches and colds
- Toothache
- Stimulant
- Dysentery
- Cystitis
- Urethritis
- Gastric spasm
- Hysteria
- Laryngitis
- Dermatitis

Safety: General regarded as safe.

Hazards: Essential oils high in 1,8-cineole can cause CNS and breathing problems in young children. Contraindications: Do not apply to or near the face of infants or children.

Calendula

Calendula officinalis

Historical successes of using this **essential oil** and **carrier oil** have included:

- Ulcers of all kinds from mouth ulcers to ulcerative colitis
- Conjunctivitis
- Ear infections
- Aids liver function – so jaundice
- Nappy rash
- Cracked nipples
- Mastitis
- Eczema
- Varicose veins

- Haemorrhoids
- Abscesses
- Damaged skin especially after surgery or radiation treatment

Safety: General regarded as safe.

You can find an article on calendula at buildyourownreality.com/calendula

Chamomile Maroc or Moroccan Chamomile
Ormenis horticaulis

Historical successes of using this **essential oil** have included:

- Very gentle oil
- Relaxing, soothing and sedative
- Itchy skin
- Digestive
- Tummy upsets
- Generally calming

Safety: Generally regarded as safe.

Note: Nomenclature can be confusing here. Be very careful not to confuse Chamomile Maroc with *Moroccan Blue Chamomile, sometimes also called Moroccan Blue Tansy which is neurotoxic.* Also Tansy, (*Tancetum vulgare*) is neurotoxic too. You might see it incorrectly listed as Blue Tansy on some sites, this is a different oil again! Blue Tansy *Tanacetum Annuum* is a naturally occurring hybrid of Roman Chamomile and Chamomile matricaria which is generally regarded as safe.

Chamomile Matricaria

Chamomilla matricaria

Historical successes of using this **essential oil** have included:

- Inflammations
- Arthritis & Muscular pain
- Menstrual pain
- Headache
- Insomnia

- Nervous complaints and anxiety
- Intestinal parasites
- Colic
- Nappy rash
- Cracked nipples
- Hayfever
- Insomnia
- Haemorrhoids
- Diarrhoea
- Neuralgia
- Toothache
- Earache
- Chicken pox itching
- Eye infections and inflammation
- Conjunctivitis

Safety: Generally regarded as safe.

Chamomile matricaria is covered in far more depth in a monograph I have written not only about its history but also the extensive clinical trials being done on this oil for possible future drug usages into cancer amongst other conditions. You can download this as buildyourownreality.com/camomile/

Chamomile Roman
Anthemis nobilis

Historical successes of using this **essential oil** have included:

- This is the most anti-inflammatory of the three chamomiles and in fact of most essential oils
- Allergies
- Redness and soreness
- Very calming so good for children
- Has a tonic effect on the liver
- Irritation, either physical or emotional
- Digestive

- Diarrhoea

- Restless legs

- Swelling and oedema

- Cramps and spasms

Safety: General regarded as safe.

Cardamon

Historical successes of using this **essential oil** have included:

- Sciatica

- Coughs

- Spasms

- Abdominal pains

- Urinary retention

- Aphrodisiac

- Digestive problems esp. heartburn

- Flatulence

- Diarrhoea

Safety: General regarded as safe.

NB: Skin irritant. Do not use on the face of young children because of high levels of 1;8 cineole known to cause central nervous system and respiratory complaints.

Caraway

Carum carvi

Historical successes of using this **essential oil** have included:

- Loss of appetite
- Indigestion
- Flatulence
- Intestinal parasites
- Vertigo
- Painful periods
- Lactation

Safety: General regarded as safe.

Carrot Seed

Daucus carota

Historical successes of using this **essential oil** have included:

- Tonic for the liver and gall bladder
- Ulcerative conditions
- Tones the skin and restores elasticity
- Cleans the skin of pollutants

Safety: General regarded as safe.

Do not use in pregnancy or whilst breast feeding

Cassia

Cinnamomum cassia

Historical successes of using this **essential oil** have included:

- Antifungal
- Toenail fungus
- Diarrhoea

- Viral and bacterial infections

- Kidney infections and urinary tract infections

- Ringworm and intestinal worms

Safety: Extremely irritant oil. Very burning to the skin and mucous membranes, I would avoid this oil on the skin at all costs. Contraindicated in pregnancy. Inhibits blood clotting. Must not be used with blood clotting or diabetes medications, or at time of surgery.

Catnip

Nepeta cataria

Historical successes of using this **essential oil** have included:

- Insect repellent, especially important in deterring mosquitos

- Sedative oil

- Cramps and spasms in particular IBS and colic

- Astringent – tightens the skin so useful in skin care, cellulite and dieting!

- Shaking limbs, dystonia, tremors, Parkinson's (but not epilepsy. See safety)
- Tightens the gums

More in depth report available here:

Safety: Mildly neurotoxic and so not suitable for use with epilepsy. May be psychotropic.

Cedarwood Atlas
Cedrus atlantica

Historical successes of using this **essential oil** have included:

- Bronchial
- Urinary tract infections and problems
- Cystitis and urinary tract infections
- Breaks down mucous
- Mildly astringent
- Acne – in particular in males (masculine fragrance so good for skin care)

- Dandruff

- Tonic for the entire body

- Regulates menstruation.

- Reduces stress and tension

Safety: Generally regarded as safe.

Because of its action on the reproductive system, I would also suggest do not use in pregnancy.(EA)

Cedarwood Virginian

Juniperus Virginia

The eagle-eyed of you will have noticed, despite the similar names, these come from trees from entirely different families. That said, their properties are unusually similar too.

Similar, but perhaps stronger than atlas

Historical successes of using this **essential oil** have included:

- Muscular aches and pains, especially resulting from exercise and training; seems to tone them.

- Decongestant to the veins so: Haemorrhoids, varicose veins etc.

Safety – Generally regarded as safe.

NB Do not use in pregnancy, or if there is a possibility of becoming pregnant (EA)

Celery Seed
Apium graveolens

Historical successes of using this **essential oil** have included:

- Rids the body of toxins so is probably the best treatment for gout
- Cleanses the liver and gall bladder
- Tonic to the digestive system
- Excellent skin cleanser

Safety: Generally regarded as safe. However use of old oils should be avoided because of threat of sensitisation from old oils.

Cinnamon Bark

Complex oil as Cassia oil is sometimes labelled as cinnamon bark. This profile however is for *cinnamomum verum*.

Safety: High risk of skin sensitisation. Irritating to the skin and mucous membranes. Inhibits blood clotting. This oil should be avoided.

Cinnamon Leaf

Cinnamomum verum

Historical successes of using this **essential oil** have included:

- Infections
- Bronchitis
- Arthritis
- Rheumatism

Safety: Very slight dermal irritant, so do not use on sensitive skin. Should be avoided by any patients who have platelet problems such as haemophilia or who are taking blood thinning medication such as heparin, warfarin or enoxoparin. Use in a maximum dilution of 0.6%

Clary Sage

Salvia sclarea

Historical successes of using this **essential oil** have included:

- Brings about a euphoric state
- Drowsy and sedative
- Muscle relaxant
- Asthma – relaxes the bronchial tubes
- Tension migraines
- Cramps
- Colicky pain and digestive problems
- Menstrual cramps
- Scanty and missing periods
- Aphrodisiac

Safety: Encourages contractions in labour and so is useful when labour is confirmed by a midwife, otherwise avoid in pregnancy.

Clove Bud

Syzygium aromanticum

Historical successes of using this **essential oil** have included:

- Memory deficiency
- Contagious disease
- Flatulence
- Dyspepsia
- Stomach cramps
- Pulmonary infections
- Toothache

Safety: Moderate dermal irritant, so use only in small dilutions. Should be avoided by any patients who have platelet problems such as haemophilia or who are taking blood thinning medication such as heparin, warfarin or enoxoparin.

Coriander Seed

Coriandrum sativum

Historical successes of using this **essential oil** have included:

- Digestive
- Flatulence
- Anorexia
- Analgesic
- Neuralgia
- Rheumatism
- Nervous debility
- Rheumatic pain

Safety: Generally regarded as safe.

Cumin

Cuminum cyminum

Historical successes of using this **essential oil** have included:

- Antispasmodic

- Digestive

- Tonic

- Stimulant, especially to the heart and nervous systems

- Aphrodisiac

Safety: Moderate risk of phototoxicity. Do not use for 12 hours before exposure to bright sunlight or going on a sunbed. Use in dilutions of less than 0.4%

Cypress

Cupressus sempervirens

Historical successes of using this **essential oil** have included:

- Refreshing

- Diuretic so flushes the system out

- Menstrual problems and pain and of course bloating

- Menopausal symptoms and pain

- Headaches causes from too much TV, computer or office static

- Astringent so cleansing to oily skin and hair

Safety: Generally regarded as safe. High risk of oxidation, so do not use old oils.

Damiana
Turnera diffusa

Historical successes of using this **essential oil** have included:

- Über – Aphrodisiac

- More an oil for marital sex than liaisons because it has a bonding quality to it

- Very relaxing

- Releases sexual tension in the pelvis

- Helps with stamina

- Digestive

- Menstrual problems

Safety: Generally regarded as safe.

There is an in depth article about damiana at buildyourownreality.com/damiana

Dill

- Digestion
- Stomach cramps
- Bloating,
- Constipation,
- Heartburn,
- Indigestion

Safety: Generally regarded as safe.

Elemi

Canarium luzonicum

Historical successes of using this **essential oil** have included:

Again this has similar qualities to frankincense

- Brings elasticity to sagging skin and so treats wrinkles
- Tightening for conditions such as cellulite
- Respiratory- rather than clearing it is opening...
- Asthma, emphysema, COPD

Safety: Generally regarded as safe. Old and oxidised oils can cause skin sensitisation.

Eucalyptus
Eucalyptus globulus

One of the most important oils in the box! There are in fact many different types of eucalyptus each with different properties. I shall be writing a paper on the family and its different members early next year.

Historical successes of using this **essential oil** have included:

- Decongestant...obviously
- Anti-bacterial and anti viral

- Respiratory infections
- Tonic to the liver
- Mouth wash for oral bacteria
- Measles

Safety: Generally regarded as safe. Because of high levels of 1,8 cineole, which can cause depression of the central nervous system and breathing difficulties, do not use on children's faces.

Fennel
Foeniculum vulgare

Historical successes of using this **essential oil** have included:

- Carminative
- Digestive
- Nausea
- Flatulence
- Indigestion
- Hiccups

- Colic
- Stimulates appetite
- Diuretic
- Urinary tract infections
- Prevents kidney stones
- Cellulite
- Stimulates oestrogen
- Stimulates lactation
- Pulmonary disease
- Intestinal parasites
- Nervous vomiting

Hazards: Drug interaction; reproductive hormone modulation; potentially carcinogenic, based on estragole content; may inhibit blood clotting; skin sensitization if oxidized. Contraindications (all routes): Pregnancy, breastfeeding, endometriosis, estrogen-dependent cancers, children under five years of age. Cautions: Diabetes medication, anticoagulant medication, major surgery, peptic ulcer, haemophilia, other bleeding disorders

Fir, silver

Abies alba

Historical successes of using this **essential oil** have included:

- Aches and pains from repetitive strain
- Bursitis
- Frozen shoulder
- Over exercise
- Cartillage inflammation
- Arthritis
- Sinus congestion
- Breaks a fever
- Opens the airways so useful for asthma and wheezing
- Airborne bacteria – use in a spray

Safety: Generally regarded as safe. High probability of oxidation which can cause skin sensitisation. Do not use old oils.

Frankincense

Boswelia carterii

Historical successes of using this **essential oil** have included:

- Skin preservative – resin was used to embalm mummies!
- Very dry and mature skin
- Tendonitis
- Respiratory complaints – opens the airways
- Slows down breathing so hyperventilation
- Very calming to anxiety

Safety: Generally regarded as safe.

High probability of oxidation, so do not use old oils.

Galangal

Alpinia galangal

Historical successes of using this **essential oil** have included:

- Very similar uses to its cousin ginger, but probably gentler I think.

- Tummy upsets

- Nausea, especially travel sickness

- Warming

- Lustily aphrodisiac!

- Slightly antifungal

- Regulates periods

Safety: Generally regarded as safe.

Because of the effects on the reproductive system, this oil is best avoided in pregnancy.(EA)

Galbanum

Ferula gummosa

Historical successes of using this **essential oil** have included:

- Another embalming oil from the caches of Ancient Egypt

- Incredible skin healer, especially of ulcerated skin

- Relaxes, tense overtired muscles (especially from emotional stress)

- Wrinkles

- Helps skin renewal

- Mature skin that is oily or acne prone

- Healing to scar tissue

Safety: Generally regarded as safe.

I wrote an in depth article for the 2010 copy of Aromatherapy Thymes, the professional Journal of the International Federation of Aromatherapists about Galbanum. You can access it at buildyourownreality.com/galbanum/ if you would like to add it to your reference files.

Geranium Egypt
Pelargonium graveolens

Historical successes of using this **essential oil** have included:

- Hormonal balancer – menopausal, PMS and teenagers!!!

- Depression

- Nervous tension

- Circulatory

- Haemorrhoids

- Prostate problems

- Dry skin and broken capillaries

- This oil has an in depth profile written here

Safety: Generally regarded as safe.

There is much excitement about developments into how geranium oil may be able to help recovery from breast cancer after chemotherapy amongst other conditions. I have written an in depth monologue about this. You can download this at *buildyourownreality.com/geranium*

Geranium Bourbon

Pelargonium roseum

Historical successes of using this **essential oil** have included:

Again, similar properties but this time the oil had that lovely rosy scent. Rich and full bodied.

This would be my choice for depression over the others.

Safety: Generally regarded as safe.

Ginger

Zingiber officinale

Historical successes of using this **essential oil** have included:

Any condition where the body is struggling to cope with moisture so:

- Runny nose
- Catarrh
- Chesty cough
- Fluid retention
- Cellulite
- Diarrhoea

As well as:

- Rheumatic pain
- Stomach cramps

- Nausea
- Impotence
- Sore throat
- Tonsilitis

Safety: Generally regarded as safe.

Gingergrass

Cymbopogon martini

This relative of lemongrass is sunshine on a snotty, rainy day!

Historical successes of using this **essential oil** have included:

- Uplifting
- Chases away fatigue
- Refreshing
- Sinus congestion
- Throat allergies
- Antifungal – athletes foot toe nail infections

Safety: Generally regarded as safe. High levels of oxidation which can cause skin sensitisation with this oil. Do not use old oils.

Grapefruit

Citrus paradise

Historical successes of using this **essential oil** have included:

- Fresh, zingy, uplifting note
- Stimulates appetite
- Tonic for the liver
- Breaks down fat
- Stimulant to the circulation and lymphatic systems
- Tones and cleanses the skin, especially helpful to oily skins

Safety: Phototoxic so do not use less than 30 mins before going out into the sunshine. This oil is contraindicated with HIV medicines and also any calcium channel blocking medications

such as heparin, warfarin or clexane. Again, high risk of oxidation, so do not use old oils.

Helichrysum

Helichrysum angustifolium (or there is also *italicum* on sale which is also helichrysum)

One of the most useful oils because it is an overall tonic and fortifies any physical mix. You might also see this listed as Everlasting or Immortelle. Everlasting is a great description because it builds resilience and stamina. If something is sluggish and stagnant this is a good oil to move it.

Historical successes of using this **essential oil** have included:

- Antispasmodic – cramps, coughs, tummy aches
- Prevents blood thickening, so useful in case of high cholesterol
- Clotting and painful menstruation
- Clears phlegm and congestion
- Digestive – sluggish

- Circulation- sluggish

- Congested and impacted skin, helps with new skin regeneration

Safety: Generally regarded as safe. Slight risk of skin irritation. Do not use in dilutions exceeding 0.5%

Hinoki

Chamaecyparis obtuse

This is - from a Japanese Cypress. It is a treasured and well loved oil in Japan but the wood from which it is distilled is now protected. New sources are emerging from Taiwan and there is a contact at the back of the book if you would like to acquire some, as it is difficult to source in the UK yet. The company, Aquagreen, manufacture figurines from the wood and then produce essential oil from the chippings.

Historical uses of this **essential oil** have included:

- Anti-inflammatory

- Pain relieving

- Cooling to conditions that feel like they are burning or hot

- Extremely sedative and meditative and particularly useful for yoga

- Insect repellent (it is so useful for buildings because termites do not like it)

- Odour elimination

- Prevents mould and bacteria.

- Fungicidal

- Candida

- Athletes foot

Safety – Generally regarded as safe.

Hyssop

Hyssopus officinalis

Historical successes of using this **essential oil** have included:

- Chest infections

- Catarrh

- Respiratory difficulties

- Gargle for sore throats

- Bruising

- Aids mental clarity

Safety: Contraindicated in cases of high blood pressure and epilepsy, fever or pregnancy. Do not use on young children. Tisserand and Young cite Hyssop (linanool) as having none of these contraindications. Do not exceed dilutions of 0.3%

Inula

Inula graveolens

(There is a cousin, *Inula helinium,* but avoid this one as it is extremely irritating to the skin)

If I went on Desert Island Discs and they said I could only take one oil with me, this would be mine. I have very sensitive respiratory system after having suffered a blood clot in my lungs. Inula is my salvation when I start barking like a dog!!!

It is very strong, use only in very small dilutions.

Historical successes of using this **essential oil** have included:

- Tonic to the respiratory system

- Opens up the airways in wheezing and asthmatic conditions

- Breaks down congestion and catarrh

- Reduces coughing

- Increases immunity (in fact Shirley Price recommends it for treatment of HIV/Aids patients)

Safety: Very harsh dermal irritant. Use only in very small dilutions and not a great idea to put this one in the bath. Please do not use in pregnancy.

Jasmine
Jasminum officinale

Historical successes of using this **absolute** have included:

- Hot dry skin

- Uterine tonic so any gynaecological problems pertaining to the womb

- Endometriosis

- Wonderful skin healer

- Strengthens contractions in childbirth (do not use until labour is confirmed by the midwife)

- Soothes depression especially if related to anxiety

- Aphrodisiac – helps with both frigidity and impotence

- Sore throats & Laryngitis

- Urinary tract infections

Safety: Generally regarded as safe.

Do not use in pregnancy except in labour which has been confirmed as established. Its uterine contraction effect could expel the foetus. Slight risk of skin sensitisation (presumably because of known adulterants) Do not exceed suggested dilution of 0.7%

Juniper
Juniperus communis

Historical successes of using this **essential oil** have included:

- Diuretic so any condition where water is being retained

- It clears waste products from the body

- Antiseptic and astringent: Urinary infections

- Cellulite

- Cystitis

- Acne – especially useful for boys as it has a more masculine fragrance

- Loss of appetite

- Painful periods

- Breaks down uric acid crystals so rheumatism, arthritis gout

- Useful oil for dogs and cats. Prevents fleas and tic and also canker.

Safety: Generally regarded as safe. High risk of oxidation and so do not use old oils which could lead to skin sensitisation.

Kanuka

Kunzea ericoides or it is more recently been reclassified to Leptospernum ericoides. Either labelling on a bottle would be correct but may, I suppose, date the time of extraction potentially.

Very similar to tea tree.

Historical successes of using this **essential oil** have included:

- Antifungal
- Antiparasitic
- Astringent to the skin
- Cleansing and respiratory
- Its most important function is antiviral and in boosting the immune system in times of infection

Safety: Generally regarded as safe. High risk of oxidation and so do not use old oils which could lead to skin sensitisation.

Labdanum
Cistus ladaniferus

Historical successes of using this **essential oil** have included:

More often used in perfumery than aromatherapy, but it has two very potent uses

- A lovely oil for wrinkles
- Deeply sedative and relaxing – ideal for meditation

Safety: Generally regarded as safe.

Lavandin

Lavandula hybrida

Lavandin is a perfect example of a lavender chemotype. It is a cross between two species of lavender *Lavendula vera* and *Lavendula latifolia* , and because the resulting scent is much stronger and pungent is usually the "lavender" of choice for the soap industry.

It is more of a clinical oil than lavender. Its high camphor content means it is much more antiseptic. On the downside this makes it unsuitable for treating burns.

Otherwise take lavenders properties and work from there. Use only in small dilutions though, because of the camphor component.

Safety: Generally regarded as safe. Moderate risk of skin sensitisation. Tisserand and Young suggest not to exceed dilutions of 0.03% for dermal use as this is the highest dilution guaranteed not to cause an effect.

Lavender

Lavandula angustifolia

Historical successes of using this **essential oil** have included:

- Ability to restore balance: whether to mind, body or to spirit.
- Cleansing wounds
- Colds, coughs, catarrh and sinusitis, influenza
- Important treatment for burns - can be used neat.
- Headache, massage onto the temples
- Muscular pain
- Rheumatism and arthritis
- Menstrual pain or scanty periods

- Palpitations and reduces high blood pressure.
- Acne especially with bergamot - inhibits the flow of sebum.
- Depression and hysteria
- Insomnia

Safety – Generally regarded as safe. *Tisserand and Young suggests not to exceed dilutions of 1% for dermal use as this is the highest dilution guaranteed not to cause an effect. This seems over cautious to me.*

There is a monograph for Lavender including details of blending, history and information of clinical trials into lavender for future drug possibilities. You can download it at buildyourownreality.com/lavender

Lemon
Citrus limonum

Historical successes of using this **essential oil** have included:

- Stimulates creation of white corpuscles
- Infection
- Wounds
- Bronchitis and influenza
- Gastric infections
- Reduces temperature
- Bactericidal
- Counteracts acidity in the body (paradoxically!)
- Cooling and refreshing
- Chilblains
- Insect bites
- Snake bites
- Tonic for the liver and pancreas
- Rheumatism and arthritis
- Circulation

- Varicose veins

- High blood pressure

- Warts, corns and verrucae (use neat on the affected area, dab with a cotton bud)

- Gallstones

- Seborrhoea

- Brittle nails

- Tender feet

- Whitens teeth apparently!

Safety: generally regarded as safe. Risk of skin sensitisation from using old or oxidised oils.

Lemon Balm
See Melissa

Lemongrass
Cymbopogon flexuosus

Historical successes of using this **essential oil** have included:

- Anti-infectious
- Fevers
- Headaches
- Antiseptic
- Deodorant
- Insect repellent: Fleas and tics.
- Refreshing
- Tired and sweaty feet

Safety: Advised to avoid in pregnancy. Has the risk of teratrogenicity, (which is the formation of birth defects). Moderate threat of skin irritation due to aldehyde content. Use in small dilution to test for sensitivity on first usage.

Lime
Citrus aurantifolia

Historical successes of using this **essential oil** have included:

- Perfect for refreshing a tired mind

- Cleanses the hair to give vibrant, lustrous locks
- Restorative
- Invigorating

Safety: Generally regarded as safe. High risk of oxidation which can lead to skin sensitisation, so do not use old or oxidised lime oil.

Linden Blossom
Tilia cordata T Parvifolia

Historical successes of using this **absolute** have included:

Again, more used in perfumery than aromatherapy.

All stress related conditions including:

- Migraine
- Insomnia
- Panic attacks
- Irritable bowel syndrome

Safety: Generally regarded as safe

Litsea Cubeba

Litsea cubeba

Historical successes of using this **essential oil** have included:

This is also sometimes listed as May Chang

Not that many physical uses but will feature heavily in my Essential Oils for the Emotions books!

- Very stimulating to fight off fatigue and lethargy
- Steadying in nervous disorders.

Safety summary Hazards: Drug interaction; tetratogenicity (birth defects); skin allergy. Cautions:

Diabetes medication, pregnancy. Cautions (dermal): Hypersensitive, diseased or damaged skin, children under 2 years of age. Maximum dermal use level: 0.8%

Mandarin

Citrus reticulate

Historical successes of using this **essential oil** have included:

- Tonic for the adrenals

- Digestive, use for burps, hiccups, nausea
- Is a very good children's remedy because it is very gentle.
- Marjoram
- Helps to free up breathing
- Asthma
- Colds – use as a steam inhalation
- Warming, analgesic, sedative
- Steadies the central nervous system
- Dilates the arteries to reduces high blood pressure
- Warming to the muscles
- Arthritis and rheumatism
- Stomach cramps
- Peristalsis
- Anxiety
- Migraine

- Respiratory spasms
- Nervous tics
- Weakness and debility

Safety: Generally regarded as safe. Do not use old or oxidised mandarin oil as it can lead to skin sensitisation

Manuka

Leptospermum scoparium

Familiar I am sure to people as the plant bees feast on to make manuka honey.

Historical successes of using this **essential oil** have included:

- Particularly important for its anti-inflammatory effects on the gut
- IBS, Crohn's, Colitis
- Anti fungal
- Antibacterial and anti-infectious
- Insect bites and stings

- Heals wounds and encourages scar tissue after surgery

Safety: Generally regarded as safe.

Marigold – see Calendula and Tagetes

Marjoram

Origanum marjorana

Historical successes of using this **essential oil** have included:

- Tonic for the Central nervous system
- Insomnia
- Migraine headaches
- Anti-spasmodic to all muscles including cardiac and pulmonary tissues
- Slightly diuretic so helpful for water retention

Safety: Generally regarded as safe.

May chang – see Litsea cubeba

Melissa

Melissa officinalis, also known as Lemon Balm

Historical successes of using this **essential oil** have included:

- Anti-allergenic so useful for hayfever etc
- Uplifting
- Anti viral
- Tonic to the liver and spleen
- Very strengthening oil to the entire system
- Is being trialled to help with cognitive impairment in dementia (use with lavender)

Safety: Advised to avoid in pregnancy. Has the risk of tetragenicity, which is the formation of birth defects. Moderate threat of skin irritation due to aldehyde content. Use in small dilution to test for sensitivity on first usage.

Mint – see peppermint and spearmint

Myrrh

Commiphora myrhha

Historical successes of using this **essential oil** have included:

- Incredible skin healer, and was used in the embalming process of mummification
- Cuts through congestion, so use for catarrh and chesty coughs
- Relaxing to smooth muscle tissues
- Uterine stimulant so useful after childbirth
- Deeply relaxing and uplifting

Safety: because of its uterine actions, not safe to use in pregnancy except in labour declared to be established by a midwife. Do not use whilst breast feeding.

I have written a far more in depth monograph about myrrh oil containing history, blending notes and details of clinical trials and experimentation into myrrh for possible future drug treatments. You can download it for free at buildyourownreality.com/myrrh

Myrtle

Myrtus communis

Historical successes of using this **essential oil** have included:

- Coughs and colds especially for small children
- Soothing for babies and children who are upset
- Respiratory infections
- Asthma, bronchitis, emphysema
- Balancing to the ovaries and thyroid

Safety: Generally regarded as safe. Do not use with diabetes medication as there are possible carcinogenic results. Use maximum dilution of 1.9%

There is a further article on myrtle here.

Neroli

Citrus aurantium

Historical successes of using this **absolute** have included:

- Antidepressant

- Antispasmodic

- Sedative

- Anxiety

- Skin care (especially for dry, sensitive, more mature skins)

- Aphrodisiac in that it relieves nervous tension

- Cardiac spasm

- Chronic diarrhoea

- Nervous dyspepsia

Safety: Generally regarded as safe.

Niaouli

Maleleuca quinquinervia, sometimes also extracted from maleleuca viridiflora

Historical successes of using this **essential oil** have included:

- Cousin of cajeput, but in many ways is much gentler

- Very easy in the mucous membranes

- Excellent for cleansing skin wounds, especially if they have dirt in them
- Burns
- Stimulates tissue healing
- Antiseptic – especially useful for acne
- Respiratory tract infections
- Influenza
- Pneumonia
- Whooping cough
- Rhinitis
- Sinusitis
- Urinary tract infections
- Intestinal parasites

Safety: Generally regarded as safe. Do not use on children's faces as it contains high levels of 1,8 cineole which can depress the central nervous system and cause respiratory complaints.

Nutmeg

Myristica fragrans

Historical successes of using this **essential oil** have included:

- Rheumatic pain
- Stimulating to the circulation and heart
- Supports the pituitary gland
- Diarrhoea (chronic)
- Intestinal infections
- Aids digestion of greasy and starchy foods (Get the rice pudding out!!!)
- Bad breath
- Loss of appetite
- Gall stones
- Scant periods

Safety: Use in small dilutions as has been reported to be psychotropic! Do not use with the drug, Pethadine. Possibly may be carcinogenic. Not recommended for use in pregnancy. Do not exceed 5% dilution.

Olibanum

See Frankincense

Orange, bitter

Citrus aurantium

Historical successes of using this **essential oil** have included:

- Useful for the mouth
- Sore gums, ulcers etc
- Sluggish digestion
- Revives dull looking complexions
- Uplifting

Safety: mildly phototoxic. Use in dilutions of less than 0.5% if there is to be exposure to sunlight during the next 12 hours. High risk of oxidation so using old oils could lead to skin sensitisation.

Orange, sweet

Citrus sinensis

Historical successes of using this **essential oil** have included:

Cleanses stinky rooms, especially of cigarette smoke

Similar uses to above, perhaps more calming and soothing

Safety note: No threat of phototoxicity (compare bitter orange). High risk of oxidation so using old oils could lead to skin sensitisation.

Oregano

Origanum vulgare

Historical successes of using this **essential oil** have included:

- Loss of appetite
- Sluggish digestion
- Bronchitis and tickly coughs
- Asthma
- Chronic rheumatism
- Muscular pain

- Absence of periods

Safety: Generally regarded as safe.

However Tisserand and Young also lists hazards to be aware of:

"Drug interaction; inhibits blood clotting; embryotoxicity; skin irritation (low risk); mucous membrane irritation (moderate risk). Contraindications (all routes): Pregnancy, breastfeeding. Cautions (dermal): Hypersensitive, diseased or damaged skin, children under two years of age. Cautions: anticoagulant medication, major surgery, peptic ulcer, haemophilia, other bleeding disorders. Maximum dermal use level: 1.1%"

Palma Rosa
Cymbopogon martinii

Historical successes of using this **essential oil** have included:

- Hydrating
- Stimulating
- Balances sebum production

Safety: Generally regarded as safe.

Patchouli

Pogostemon cablin

Historical successes of using this **essential oil** have included:

- Dry skin
- Skin regeneration
- Athletes foot
- Fluid retention
- Aphrodisiac
- Acne

Safety: Generally regarded as safe.

Inhibits blood clotting, so do not use whilst on blood thinning medication, prior to major surgery, or if there is a clotting disorder such as haemophilia.

Peppermint

Mentha piperata

Historical successes of using this **essential oil** have included:

- Stimulating (do not use before bed, or you will never sleep).

- Reviving and refreshing, clears the head

- Lovely and cooling, especially for tired feet

- Reduces heat, so fevers, inflamed skin etc

- Tonic to the liver

- Digestive, heart burn, indigestion

- Stimulates bile.

Safety: Generally regarded as safe. Not suitable for use in pregnancy.

In high dilutions has a mild threat of neurotoxicity. Stimulates the heart, so there is a risk of fibrillation If using on a person with epilepsy or with a heart complaint, consider homeopathic dose. Irritating to the mucous membranes. Not suitable for patients with G6PD deficiency.

Petitgrain
Citrus aurantium amara

Historical successes of using this **essential oil** have included:

- Similar to neroli (it comes from the same tree, this is the leaves and twigs sitting around neroli's blossom)
- Sedative and stimulant – so might possibly make it difficult to sleep
- Deodorant

Safety: Generally regarded as safe.

Pimento

Pimenta officinalis

Historical successes of using this **essential oil** have included:

Also known as all-spice

More for emotional uses really but..

- Rheumatism and muscular aches and pains
- Add into diffuser blends for chest congestion

Safety: Potentially carcinogenic due to methyleugenol content. May inhibit blood clotting, irritate the skin and mucous membrane. Tisserand and Young recommend a maximum dilution of 0.15%

Pine

Pinus sylvestris

Historical successes of using this **essential oil** have included:

- Chest infections
- Pneumonia
- Expectorant
- Pulmonary antiseptic
- Stimulating to the circulation
- Rheumatic pain
- Refreshing
- Deodorant
- Muscular pain
- Cystitis

- Prostatis
- Inflammation of the gall bladder
- Infections
- Impotence
- Rickets
- Intestinal pain

Safety: Moderate dermal irritant. (Do not use in the bath!)

Plai

Zingiber Cassumunar

- Rheumatism
- Arthritis
- Joint Pain
- Muscle Rubs
- Pain relieving and anti-inflammatory

Safety – Generally regarded as safe.

Ravensara

Ravensara aromatica

Historical successes of using this **essential oil** have included:

Pain relieving for:

- Tooth ache
- Headaches
- Muscular and joint pains
- Earache
- Reputed to be anti-allergenic – but I have not used it myself for this

Antispasmodic especially to the respiratory system.

- Asthma, bronchitis, coughs
- Expectorant – shifts catarrh and mucous
- Also leg spasms, pain in the gut from diarrhoea
- Antiviral – so useful for cleaning surfaces and treating colds and tummy bugs
- Disinfectant

- Diuretic so useful for oedema, swelling, bloating

- Rheumatic pain

- Aphrodisiac

Safety note: *May have a risk of being carcinogenic based on its estragole content. Otherwise regarded as safe.*

Rose

Rosa damascena

Historical successes of using this **essential oil** have included:

- Uterine stimulant and tonic

- Eases menstrual pain

- Helps labour

- Feeds the skin

- Aphrodisiac

- Nourishing and nurturing

- Encourages grief to recede

Safety: Avoid in pregnancy, except in confirmed established labour, because of its uterine properties.

Rose oil has been "the queen of oils" for many centuries. There is an in depth monologue investigating its history right up to the recent experiments into rose for possible future drug trials. You can download this at buildyourownreality.com/rose/

Rosemary
Rosmarinus officinalis

Historical successes of using this **essential oil** have included:

- Aids mental clarity, good for concentration and memory

Recommended for all types of nerve pain, for example:

- Sciatica
- Neuralgia
- Headache
- Migraine

- Lowers cholesterol
- Invigorating and stimulating
- Indigestion and bloating
- Constipation
- Stimulates appetite
- Improves circulation

Hair care:

- Dandruff
- Stimulates the scalp
- Use as a final rinse for glassy dark hair

Safety data: Not safe to use in pregnancy and is also neurotoxic. Do not use with high blood pressure or epilepsy. Because of 1,8 cineole content, do not use on children's faces.

Rosewood

Aniba Rosaeodora var. amazonia ducke also known as Rosewood

Historical successes of using this **essential oil** have included:

- Cephalic, so excellent for headaches
- Driving stress
- Antibacterial
- Tonic, but not stimulant:
- Insecticide
- Wound healing
- Increases libido
- Clears the mind and allows you to focus – particularly good for exams

Safety: Generally regarded as safe.

Sage
Salvia officinalis

Historical successes of using this **essential oil** have included:

An interesting oil which is cited on many websites as being useful for:

- Heavy sweating
- Stimulates appetites and digestion
- Muscle stiffness

However: I would replace with clary sage in blends because....

Safety: This oil causes heavy bleeding in women and has a very high level of ketones (thujone) which can lead to convulsions and also skin irritation. It is also neurotoxic. Do not use in pregnancy or in breastfeeding.

Sandalwood

There are various sandalwoods all coming from different parts of the world. *Sandalwood mysore*, potentially is a more refined version, but this is the most available version.

Santalum album

Historical successes of using this **essential oil** have included:

- Urinary Tract infections
- Pulmonary antiseptic
- Coughs, colds, bronchitis
- Sore throats
- Dry dehydrated skins
- Oily skins and acne
- Chronic diarrhoea
- Astringent
- Antiseptic
- Aphrodisiac

Safety: Generally regarded as safe.

Spearmint

Mentha spicata

Historical successes of using this **essential oil** have included:

Not that dissimilar to peppermint, spearmint has a less stimulating edge.

- Cleans wounds and ulcers and speeds healing
- Antispasmodic
- Digestive
- Flatulence
- Indigestion and heartburn
- Bloating
- Gastro-intestinal spasm
- Irregular and missing periods
- Promotes production of oestrogen
- Insecticide, especially to mosquitoes

Safety: Generally regarded as safe. Very low risk of skin sensitisation. Tisserand and Young suggest not to use in dilutions of more than 1.7%

Spikenard

Nardostachys jatamansi

Historical successes of using this **essential oil** have included:

- Extremely sedative and analgesic
- Use for any extreme pain
- Circulatory, varicose veins, thread veins, haemorrhoids
- Digestive pain, colic, nausea and indigestion

Safety: Generally regarded as safe.

Tagetes

Tagetes minuta

Historical successes of using this **essential oil** have included:

- Anti parasitic and insecticide so fleas, nits and other crawlies
- Antifungal, athletes foot, nail infections, candida, mallesazzia
- Eczema

- Dermatitis
- Psoriasis
- Sedative to the nervous and digestive systems.

Safety: Can cause photosensitisation and also skin irritation. Is thought to be potentially carcinogenic and inhibits blood clotting. Should not be used in concentrations of more than 0.01%

Tangerine

Citrus tangerine

Historical successes of using this **essential oil** have included:

- Gentle!
- Digestive for tummy upsets
- Constipation
- Stimulates circulation
- Very cleansing to the lymphatic system
- Swelling, bloating, cellulite

- Liver tonic

Safety: Generally regarded as safe. Avoid using old or oxidised oils as they can lead to skin sensitisation.

Tarragon
Artemisia dracunculus

Historical successes of using this **essential oil** have included:

- Stimulates appetite
- Specifically thought to be effective for anorexia

NB:. Neurotoxic. This is a harmful oil to use in therapy as it is thought to be carcinogenic and toxic to the liver. The oil should be avoided in pregnancy and epilepsy in particular. It is however extremely useful to use in a diffuser, or of course the herb could be added to food. Maximum dilution suggested by Tisserand and Young is 0.1%

Tea Tree
Maleleuca alternifolia

Historical successes of using this **essential oil** have included:

Safety: Generally regarded as safe. Oils or oxidised oils may cause skin sensitisation. Maximum dilution suggested by Tisserand and Young is 15%

In my opinion the monograph on tea tree is the most fascinating of all of them. It shows how tea tree was preparing and developing into a medicine for skin cancer as long ago as twenty years past. This was picked up and predicted by a clairvoyante. Download the monograph for free at: buildyourownreality.com/teatree/

Terebinth

Pinus palastris

Historical successes of using this **essential oil** have included:

- Increases circulation and is analgesic to connective tissue so:
- Tendonitis
- Bursitis
- Frozen shoulder
- Gout

- Neuralgia

- Good for coughs and colds

- Antiseptic to the urinary tract – cystitis, urethritis

- Stems the flow of blood in nose bleeds and haemophilia

NB dermal irritant so do not use in skin in strong dilution. It has been found that irritation is usually caused by oxidation, always try to use the freshest oil you can find. Inhalation of large amounts of terebinth can lead to asthmatic effects. Neurotoxic; avoid in epilepsy or pregnancy.

Thyme
Thymus vulgaris

Historical successes of using this **essential oil** have included:

- Sluggish digestion

- Antiseptic for gastric infections

- Intestinal worms

- Pulmonary disinfectant

- Coughs and colds

- Urinary tract infections

- Low blood pressure

- Stimulates circulation

- Use for people who are fatigued, depressed and lethargic

- Rheumatic pain

- Antiviral

- Anaemia

- Illnesses from chills

Safety: Moderate dermal irritant so do not use on sensitive or damaged skins and bet to avoid use on young children. May inhibit blood clotting. Not suitable for use in pregnancy.

Tuberose

Polianthes Tuberosa

Historical successes of using this **absolute** have included:

- Sex, sex, sex!

- Alleviates frigidity

- Raises libido

- Alleviates impotence

- Very relaxing and warming

- Also sedative to the respiratory tract

Safety: Generally regarded as safe. Moderate risk of skin sensitisation, do not use on hyper-sensitive or damaged skins, or on children under 2.

I wrote a very in depth paper on Tuberose for the New Zealand Register of Holistic Therapists. You can access this at secrethealer/tuberose

Valerian
Valeriana Officinalis

Historical successes of using this **essential oil** have included:

The ultimate relaxing oil. Use for anything that seems to have no off switch, but only in small dilutions and do not mix with alcohol, you can pretty much guarantee nightmares.

- Restless leg syndrome
- Hyperactivity
- ADD / ADHD
- Grinding teeth,
- Depression and anxiety
- Tension headache
- Insomnia

Safety: Generally regarded as safe.

Vertivert

Vetivera zizanoides

Historical successes of using this **essential oil** have included:

- Relaxing, a gentler, more sultry version of valerian
- Restless leg syndrome
- Hyperactivity
- ADD / ADHD

- Grinding teeth,
- Depression and anxiety
- Tension headache
- Insomnia
- Muscular complaints
- Where valerian is more physical, vertivert is more emotionally relaxing
- Aphrodisiac

Safety: Generally regarded as safe.

Violet Leaf
Viola odorata

Historical successes of using this **absolute** have included:

- Antiseptic
- Sensitive skin
- Analgesic

- Insomnia

Safety: Generally regarded as safe.

Wintergreen
Gaultheria yunnanensis

When I first qualified this oil was categorised as toxic because there had been deaths associated with one of the primary constituents methyl salicylate. Natural wintergreen is 98% methyl salicylate, a natural occurring compound which is extremely analgesic. It is found in many liniments and even toothpastes for its minty taste. In clinical trials 7g of the constituent was found to be 300 times more pain- relieving than aspirin. Hidden from view, in so many products, it is easy to lose track of how much is being absorbed into the body. At these levels the constituent is fairly benign, but the levels in essential oil were enough for aromatherapy authorities to consider it a danger to use therapeutically.

Adding to the confusion is, many oils labelled as wintergreen, rather than being in their natural state, are thought to be synthetic copies made of pure methyl salicylate.

In addition to anyone suffering from blood clotting disorders, patients with ADD and ADHD are also thought to have a very high sensitivity to salicylates.

The properties of this **essential oil** are:

- Very cooling

- Pain relieving because it contains high concentration of methyl salicylate

- Colds and asthma

- Mentally stimulating and clearing

For clarity here I have copied and pasted directly from Tisserand and Young. I still maintain here though, please do not take essential oils orally.

Safety: Hazards: Drug interaction; inhibits blood clotting; toxicity; high doses are teratogenic.

Contraindications (all routes): Anticoagulant medication, major surgery, haemophilia, other bleeding disorders (Box 7.1). Pregnancy, breastfeeding, children. People with salicylate sensitivity (often applies in ADD/ ADHD). Maximum dermal use level: 2.4%. The risks of systemic toxicity are heightened by application onto damaged skin.

Yarrow
Achillea millefolium

Historical successes of using this **essential oil** have included:

- Extremely sedative and analgesic
- Allergies
- Any kind of pain relief
- Insomnia

Safety: In strong dilutions is neurotoxic and so should not be used in cases of epilepsy.

Hazards: Drug interaction; slight neurotoxicity. Maximum dermal use level: 8.6%

Ylang Ylang
Cananga odorata

The properties of this **essential oil** are:

- Slows heartbeat
- Palpitations
- Over rapid breathing
- Fright
- Anxiety
- High blood pressure
- Balanced the skin
- Calming and relaxing
- Aphrodisiac

Safety: Moderate risk of skin sensitisation. Tisserand and Young suggest as miaximum dilution of 0.8% and to avoid use on very young children.

Chapter 8 Oils for the systems

I have grouped oils which influence certain systems together. I find this useful if a blend is not working as I had hoped and want to see what other oils might have the same effect. It sometime helps to add more oils with the same actions to give a blend more oomph!

Pick an oil from the list and check back to the notes on the oil to ensure the correct desired outcome. Ylang ylang and thyme are both listed under circulation for their effects, for example but thyme raises it and ylang ylang lowers it. Get the wrong one and you could be in very deep water.

Respiratory System

Angelica seed, basil, cardamom, eucalyptus, ravensara, hyssop, inula, myrtle, tea tree, niaouli, ravensara, pine.

Urinary system

Jasmine, juniper, cypress, cedarwood atlas, benzoin, myrrh, fennel, bergamot, cypress, sandalwood, ginger.

Digestive System

Angelica, star anise, anise, black pepper, cardamom, caraway, carrot, clove, coriander, fennel, galangal, grapefruit, mandarin, thyme, neroli, tangerine, tarragon.

Reproductive system

Angelica, caraway, clary sage, cypress, damiana, rose, myrrh, patchouli

Aphrodisiac

Agarwood, damiana, sandalwood, jasmine, rose, cumin, neroli, tuberose, patchouli, sandalwood, ylang ylang

Lymphatic system

Elemi, fennel, juniper, cypress, ginger, grapefruit

Immunity and infection

Elemi, cajuput, niaouli, tea tree, ravensara, manuka, kanuka, cinnamon

Circulatory System

Angelica, holy basil, black pepper, cumin, galangal, geranium, ginger, helichrysm, lemon, nutmeg, thyme, spikenard, terebinth, ylang ylang

Muscular System and connective tissues

Angelica, star anise, bay, birch, cedarwood Virginian, celery, cumin, silver fir, frankincense, ginger, juniper, thyme, myrtle, pine, nutmeg, terebinth

Skin

Elemi, benzoin, myrrh, bay, birch, cade, carrot, cedarwood, celery, angelica, frankincense, galbanum, geranium, helichrysm, jasmine, labdanum, rose, lavender, calendula, sandalwood, cardamom, neroli, palma rosa, patchouli

Nervous system – Physical

Anise, holy basil, clary sage, clove, rosemary, lavender, chamomile, spikenard, yarrow

Mentally clearing

Basil, clove, rosemary, rosewood

Chapter 9 - Essential Oil Recipes Designed by Professional Aromatherapists

How you use essential oils is very much a personal thing. You will come to find you have an affinity with some oils, and pretty much ignore other oils. You will also find your own way of blending oils, not least because you will aim for slightly different effects from the oils from the next blender. For example, you might treat Irritable Bowel Syndrome by looking for oils that specifically balance the digestive system, another blender might aim for a top, middle and base mix of oils for diarrhoea and then also make a contrasting blend for constipation. The next blender might aim to address the stress and emotions that cause the flare up. None of these are wrong, they are simply different and work to the strengths of the aromatherapist.

That is where the magic lives!

In the next section, other therapists have been extremely generous and submitted the favourite blends they use in their practices. Each is a specialist in a certain field so you are going wonderful insights into how a professional works. Inevitably, most also include emotional and spiritual aspects into their treatments to get a perfect balance for their patients. You can delve further into understanding these aspects more in my book

Essential Oils for the Mind Body Spirit - The Holistic Medicine of Clinical Aromatherapy .

I decided not to edit this section to extensively, and leave the words of each therapist intact because the phraseology each uses to describe the oils and their processes really portrays not just their personalities but their passions for their craft. Some are very matter of fact about the clinical aspects of their oils whilst others bask in the wonder of the luxury of it all. I love the diversity of language it contains.

I have created a directory at the back of the book which will give you more information about each of the therapists and their practices, as well as other modalities of therapies they use. The vibrancy of difference in that section is enchanting.

Best of all are generous discounts some of them have offered for training, treatments and products so if you are looking to acquire amazing skin care, beautiful handmade perfumes, get some training in our art or of course get a massage....look no further. It is a complementary medicine shopping bonanza. Do make sure you take a look.

But first let me introduce you to each of the therapists and the beautiful recipes they have designed.

Aphrodisiac Blend – By Annie Day of Heaven Scent Bliss

Annie has worked in a women's refuge for 4 years so she's had experience of alleviating acute stress and also volunteers at the local hospice giving end of life care. Her time spent working in an NHS Sex clinic has given her the expertise to work with individuals and couples who are experiencing difficulties with Sexual Health and Sexuality issues.

2 x patchouli

2 x ylang ylang

1 x sweet orange

Diluted in 30ml grapeseed oil.

"I've been assisting people in having a great sex life for at least 15 years and this blend has been perfected over that time span using different combinations and finally using Kinesiology muscle testing to ascertain which blends work best for 20 couples who were seeing me for sex therapy/ relationship counselling 3 years ago.

So, one of the best reasons for using Patchouli is that it is a very grounding, earthy oil and when we feel safe and secure and connected to the Earth via our Earth star we can do and achieve anything. This is good for dissolving any "performance anxiety " issues and it smells divine. It is one of the longest lasting fragrances too and once satisfying love making has happened, using this blend - just one sniff of this combination and the mind will revert back to when it last smelled this and: Hey Ho it was when you were having a sensual and erotic experience.

Ylang ylang has been used for hundreds and thousands of years as an aphrodisiac. It was highly prized by Kings and Queens in Egypt, especially as a subtle perfume that stimulates sexual and sensual desire. One of its psychological properties is that it raises our self-esteem which is all important, as once we learn to love ourselves we are able to love others and are ready for our erotic and sensual desires to become a reality ((*))

Sweet orange's delicious citrus smell stimulates our taste buds as well as our olfactory system. The colour orange is also the colour of our sacral chakra where we detoxify and receive joy and pleasure. Again, once this joyful, happy, blend has been used for an erotic and sensual experience, it is locked into our Limbic system and basically the mind will say "Where was I when I last smelled this? Oh yes! I was being pleasured", which can quadruple our capacity for pleasure next time. :0)

To blend this combination - I use a glass bowl - I give a blessing, Egyptian Sekem, to all the ingredients so that they carry the vibration of unconditional love. You could use Reiki or simply bless all the ingredients before mixing. I make batches up in 30ml and 100 ml bottles sizes.

I use subtle aromatherapy techniques, learned from Patricia Davis and Josie Donaldson which suggests that if you want a particular oil to work at its maximum efficiency; less is more. So if you use a high concentration of essential oils it will only work on your physical body, and when you use a significantly lower dilution it will work on the Mind, Body and Spirit. This saves you money, as you will be using less aromatherapy oils and it works holistically too. In a 30 ml bottle I would typically use 5 drops of essential oils, and in a 100ml bottle 15 drops so that the person gets the maximum efficacy from the blend.

I add the essential oils to the bowl first and then gently stir the grape seed carrier oil in. I use grape seed oil for all massages and blends. As the nut oils such as Sweet almond, and jojoba when applied to the skin if the person has an allergy to nuts, it could potentially still cause anaphylactic shock. Likewise with wheat germ carrier oil and wheat allergies.

I always ensure that when making up the blend I ask that it will work for the persons/ couples highest good and remind them that it is great for erotic and sensual massages and IS NOT for internal use. I recommend using organic coconut oil as a lubricant as it's got great hydration properties, smells lovely, is petrochemical free and is also a natural antifungal so stops irritations such as thrush too.

I usually give couples a guide to sensual massaging techniques suggesting effleurage strokes as these are so highly enjoyable for most people and easy to do."

For more information on how to contact Annie, see the directory.

Depression blend by Dave Jackson of Cambridge Aromatherapy.

Dave holds the Diploma in Therapeutic Massage and Clinical Aromatherapy ITHMA 2000, he has been working in the mental health field for 25 years.

25ml Almond Oil

2 drops Frankincense

2 drops Bergamot

2 Drops Vetivert

I use a blend of Frankincense, Bergamot, and Vetiver for depression. Bergamot is one of the best oils for moving stagnant Qi in the Chinese medical system. Qi is considered to be the lifeforce of the body mind and soul. Vetiver is, I have found, one of the best oils for helping to ground clients. The client I use this particular blend for, also has panic attacks, as well as suffering from depression, so this grounding aspect really helps.

Frankincense, I see as an oil to help someone whose mind is overwhelmed by a "cacophony of thoughts." (To quote from my course notes!) For a depressed client, who rather than being overwhelmed by thoughts, seems to suffer from thought poverty, I would substitute Marjoram or Rosemary. Both of these are warming oils. With Frankincense, it is also worth noting there can also the danger of getting the occasional client who has unpleasant associations due bad memories or association with church etc.

I see it as important to really consider what we want a blend to achieve, and then to pick three or more oils that **all** contribute to that function. I will also be looking to each oil, to address at least two of the problems the client comes to me with. This happens organically in nature and is reflected in another of my interests, permaculture. Each element should have multiple functions and each function should be supported by multiple elements.

I like to encourage people to try blending their own sets of oil. I feel using our own or another's favourite blend for any condition should be avoided unless we have really thought it through for the individual client and their particular needs. I see this as being analogous to the practice (that is slightly less common than it used to be) of routinely giving out antibiotics when the doctor could not even be sure that it was a bacterial rather than viral infection.

Blend for ladies of that certain age…

by Clare Ella of Clare Ella Aromatherapy

Here, Clare a wonderful experience she had treating a lady in her 50s who was feeling her age. Her symptoms were:

Mild depression/ everything feeling too much/ post-menopausal/ dry skin/ general lethargy/ stressed at work/

general aches and tiredness. This blend is interesting, because, as you will see she uses more drops of essential oil than I do.

A lady in her late fifties presented with all of the above symptoms. I tend to spend quite a while talking to a new client, getting a feel for why they've come to see me, what other ways they have tried to address their symptoms or conditions, and then looking at different families of oils/ scents that I think may be appropriate, and gauging their reaction to them. In a case like this, I am always careful to ensure that the oils I use are ones that the client has a positive reaction to. If some of the oils I suggest are ones that the client is unfamiliar with, say frankincense, benzoin or plai, I always offer them the opportunity to smell the oil before including it in a blend.

In this case, the client was feeling undervalued and misunderstood at work, she was looking after an elderly, demanding parent, was not getting much support from her partner, was feeling body conscious due to weight issues, and was not sleeping properly. She felt unable to take a deep breath and 'let go'.

After enjoying her first session the client said she would come weekly, or at least 2 weeks out of 3, and we tried different blends for the first few visits, but the one that she loved most, and she felt had by far the most beneficial effects, was the one below. She relaxed into sleep during the massages, her skin felt soft and supple, she felt as if she could open her lungs and take a full breath after a session, and better equipped to cope with what life was throwing at her.

Rose Otto (*rosa damascena*) 4 drops

Black pepper (*piper nigrum*) 7 drops

Mandarin *(citrus reticulata)* 6 drops

in 22 ml apricot kernel oil

Rose Otto – wonderful for supporting the woman within, helping one to love oneself, soothing emotional anxiety and stress and relieving depression, as well as being perfect for mature, drier skin

Black pepper – a warming, grounding oil, to stimulate the mind and energise the body, whilst boosting the immune system and easing aching muscles

Mandarin – a refreshing yet calming oil, a tonic for the digestive system which could aid fat breakdown, an aid to combat insomnia and perfect for mature skin

Combined, these three oils produce a nurturing blend which works wonderfully in a base oil such as apricot kernel, enhancing the moisturising effects.

For comparison: a couple more of the mixes that we used - depending on which were the predominant symptoms that particular day - slightly frustrated, tight chest - use the Rose sandalwood, bergamot mix, if aching muscles/ mind whirring - use the Frankincense, lime, ginger mix

Rose (*Rosa damascena*) 3 drops

Sandalwood (*Santalum album)* 6 drops

Bergamot (*Citrus bergamia*) 7 drops

In 22 mls apricot kernel base oil

NB - only used in evening sessions when the client would not be exposed to sunlight/ sunbed etc following the treatment.

Rose - as above

Sandalwood - although expensive, the aroma of few oils is as immediately soothing and deeply relaxing and calming as that of true sandalwood. Helping with mild-depression, insomnia and other stress-related/induced conditions, this wonderful oil is also very useful in skincare and blends beautifully with the other 2 oils

Bergamot - this zingy, refreshing scent - with hints of floral notes- is uplifting whilst still seeming to cool anger and ease frustrations. Its positive effects on the digestive and respiratory systems made it a perfect addition to this client's blend.

Frankincense *(Boswellia carterii)* 4 dops

Lime *(Citrus aurantifolia)* 6 drops

Ginger *(Zingiber officinalis)* 4 drops

In 20 ml apricot kernel base

Frankincense - this wonderfully grounding, calming oil justifies its connection with meditative states. Helping to relieve anxiety and stress, it also acts on the respiratory system to assist deeper breathing. Good for mature skin too!

Lime - one of my favourite citrus oils - its fresh sweetness stimulates our fatigued bodies, and seeks to chase away apathy! It cuts through the heavier frankincense, stimulating the digestive system and assisting with detoxifying. I find it a very useful addition to a blend for anyone suffering from mid-depression or stress-related conditions

Ginger - this spicy 'tonic' is probably one of my most used oils - warming and analgesic for tired and aching muscles, stimulating yet calming for the digestive system, it can help to re-vitalise and improve self-confidence.

Children's Cuts and Scrapes by Sharon Falsetto of Sedona Aromatherapy
For children up to 28 lbs*

1 oz shea butter

1 drop Roman chamomile *(Chamaemelum nobile)*

1 drop lavender *(Lavandula angustifolia)*

Mix the essential oils directly with softened shea butter; apply to the affected area.

*Do not use with new born babies, unless recommended to do so by a qualified professional. Consult a certified aromatherapist for further advice on amounts to use safely with children.

Note for Using Essential Oils with Children:

- Consult a certified aromatherapist for specific circumstances if you are unfamiliar with essential oils.
- If possible, do a patch test first. Some essential oils may cause sensitivity (in the form of itching, rash, or redness) with children.
- Store essential oil bottles away from children and always keep the top fastened securely.
- Always dilute essential oils before applying to the skin with children.
- Never use essential oils internally with children.

©2014 Sharon Falsetto

Blend for Shingles by Jill Bruce of The Apothecary
In 60mls. aqueous cream
    10 drops Mandarin (Citrus reticulata)

3 drops Chamomile Matricaria (Matricaria camomilla)
2 drops Jasmine Absolute (Jasminium officinale)
4 drops Myrrh (Commiphora myrrhis)

Rub on area which is affected by the shingles, at least 4 times daily.

Mandarin helps with hypoadrenia which is very prevalent with this condition

Chamomile Matricaria - or Chamomile Blue or German as it is more commonly known is amazingly anti inflammatory and soothing, due to the component azulene. Also is analgesic.

Jasmin Absolute will minimise the scarring caused by the rash.

Myrrh will preserve the skin, and again help reduce permanent damage.

Contra-indications: if the client is pregnant, omit the Jasmine and myrrh.
Jill's details can be found in <u>the directory</u> at the back of the book.

Pregnancy and Labour Blend by Sue Mousley of SOME Training

Sue Mousley is a qualified aromatherapist and former Chairman of the International Federation of Aromatherapists. She is works as a midwife in the NHS providing help to mums in later pregnancy as well as running her own company SOME Training which teaches First Aid, Aromatherapy in Pregnancy and Baby Massage.

Sue has very generously given us two blends which I think will transform the labours of many thousands of women. This is what Sue has to say about her blends:

I have been working as a midwife since 1987 and was involved in the first water birth at the maternity unit in which I work. This started my journey into holistic health. I then discovered aromatherapy and trained with the Jill Bruce School of Aromatherapy and went on after to integrate it into my midwifery work, after searching for information and projects similar I set up a maternity aromatherapy service within an NHS Hospital.

Initially the service was just for labour but has since grown to incorporate late pregnancy and the postnatal period as well, the blends are now produced off site by a local company to my specifications and dosage and ordered straight to the relevant departments in maternity via the pharmacy department by staff and are paid for by the hospital trust.

There is a policy in place ratified and approved by the hospital trust board and staff training to ensure safety and compliance. In order to ensure this compliance there are 2 blends for late pregnancy and labour at a 1% dosage and 1 postnatal blend at 2% dosage and women are offered the choice to use alongside conventional medication if desired.

The first pregnancy/labour blend is a massage oil:

50ml - Carrier oil base of grapeseed

4 drops Lavender

3 drops Mandarin

3 drops Roman Chamomile

I chose this combination of essential oils because they felt balanced, not only do they each have an analgesic action they also approach pain and discomfort from a different angle and work on different and deeper levels.

Lavender is particularly helpful to cleanse and sooth the spirit, relieving anger and exhaustion and balancing the central nervous system. It has a sedative effect, lowering the blood pressure and aiding the release of serotonins from the brain.

Mandarin is refreshing and uplifting but has great antispasmodic properties to help with muscular spasm and revitalises and strengthens the mind and body.

Roman Chamomile has wonderful anti-inflammatory and soothing qualities promoting relaxation it is said to give patience, peace and allays worries to calm the mind whilst easing dull muscular pain particularly in the lower back.

This blend can be used from around 36 weeks of pregnancy to aid those aches and pains particularly in the low back area which many women experience it can also give the birth partner a role to play in the preparation for labour, promoting closeness and bonding. Studies have also shown that low back massage in the late pregnancy can increase the efficiency of the uterus when labour commences, and also the endorphin releasing capacity of the mother the body's natural painkillers. It can be used for anywhere on the body the main areas of tension are the low back and the neck and shoulder area.

Bath preparation for use in labour

50ml bath base

4 drops Clary Sage

6 drops Frankincense.

It was initially an equal blend but it appeared to be too powerful at this ratio.

I chose this combination because Clary Sage is a good oil to aid nervous tension and calms panicky states because of its euphoric property, the effects of which encourage feelings of wellbeing which dissipates anxiety. Clary Sage also has the properties for toning the uterus to help it work more efficiently and is thought to accelerate labour due to its oestrogen like properties, something that was noted in a study of 8000 women at the John Ratcliffe hospital in Oxford and also the reason why the ration was adjusted in my original blend, the reasoning behind this is if labour goes too rapidly it can be detrimental by increasing the mothers anxiety and causing panic which can be counterproductive by increasing adrenaline which then slows the labour and works the opposite.

Because the smell of Clary Sage can be overpowering, I chose Frankincense which compliments it perfectly. Frankincense helps clear the lungs and can help slow and deepen breathing, producing feelings of calm and reducing anxiety. It works on the biochemical for fear and panic by blocking the flow of adrenaline and other substances and also increases endorphin production.

By soaking in a warm bath with 15 mls (or about a tablespoon full) of the blend, the effect of the water combined with the oils helps the body and mind relax so that the body is able to work effectively with the mother through the labour journey in a calm and relaxed state.

Some places do use oils in the birthing pool but we don't recommend at our unit, they usually bath before entering the pool as they need to be about 4-5cms to do this so it helps keep them relaxed to get to this point so works on a different level to the pool in its approach. As long as there are active contractions when the waters break then they are ok as there is positive pressure in the uterus, if there are no contractions and the waters break, then essential oils are not advisable in the water.

Love Potion by Rebecca Brink of Serenity Thai Bodywork
I make a Love Potion roll-on with

10 drops of Lavender

8 drops of Frankincense

4 drops of Vetiver

2-3 drops of Jasmine

24 drops of almond oil

This blend is soothing and penetrates the deepest layers of the soul and love drive. It will entice and help put you and your partner in the right mood for a deep and soulful connection. Lavender is an oil that brings balance to the body and stimulates the skin. Frankincense helps to focus your energy so you are open for connection. Vetiver adds that earthy carnal base note and eases the days stress away. Jasmine is sensual and gives us a sense of hope, happiness and warmth.

Try some on you and your partners pulse points before a playful interlude and let it deepen your connection to each other.

Blend for Enhancing Self Esteem and Self Worth by Angela McKay

Angela publishes a wonderful journal via my publishing company called the *Wise Woman's Journal*. Each day it looks at the energies at play in the universe and discusses how to harness them to make the best for your day, month and life. It encompasses everything from meditations, incenses and essential oils to stunning recipes for sabbats. It is a truly beautiful work.

This is what Angie has to say about her blend.

Base oil – sweet almond 30ml

Cardamom oil 3 drops

Sandalwood oil 3 drops

Rose oil 2 drops

My stuff is about the energies around us and the planet so my blend is developed to work with the subtle energies of the body. It is healing holistically, body mind and spirit. The oils are used to increase self-esteem and love of oneself. They work with the heart chakra, Venus and Reiki movement for the heart chakra.

Pour a small amount of the mix into the palm and rub into both hands. Sitting comfortably, focused breathing/meditation etc, place the right hand over the heart chakra (where the physical heart is) and the left hand over the solar plexus (just under the breasts). Concentrate on sending healing green energy through the whole body, drawn from the heart chakra. Let the heat of the body absorb the oils into the skin. Those into Angels can call on the healing angel of the green ray, Rapheal. Just call on 'its' help to aid in the healing process. This added to whatever other physical treatment will increase your sense of well-being and encourage a greater sense of self-worth.

Cardamom is also a love oil and can be used in blends for use with others!!

The Wise Woman's Journal will be available as a yearbook in 2015. It makes a wonderful daily tool and a stunning gift for both likeminded men and woman. For a back issue from September to get a flavour of Angie's work, visit buildyourownreality.com/wwj-back-copy/

Migraine Compress by Erica Straus of Healing Essence Massage

Erica first became interested in aromatherapy when it helped her to get off of some of the many painkillers that she took for everything from headaches to backaches. She was very ill at the time and impressed with the power of essential oils. Now she runs a thriving practice in the Bay Area of California, treating patients in her clinic and also doing home visits.

Here's what Erica says about her blend:

3 drops peppermint

3 drops rosemary

Place 3 drops each of Peppermint (Mentha piperita) and Rosemary (Rosmarinus officinalis), on a damp washcloth.

Wrap the washcloth around an icepack to make a cold compress. Use the compress on the forehead, head and neck. Frequently breathe through the washcloth to inhale the vapors. Take care not to get any essential oil in the eyes as peppermint can sting. As a long-time migraine sufferer, I have experimented with numerous oils and blends. I have found this blend and process to be very helpful, both on it's own and when combined with medication.

Migraines can increase scent sensitivity, thus many essential oils recommended for headaches are unsuitable. This blend, however, is soothing and delicious. When I'm suffering from migraines I absolutely love the cooling scent. Please note that this blend is not suitable for pregnant women, infants or young children.

James I Bandits Blend to Fight Infection – By Rebecca Totilo of Aromahut

Rebecca Park Totilo and I have been friends for about 2 years now and she constantly amazes me with her wealth of knowledge about the historical aspects of essential oils.

This is what Rebecca has to say about her blend:

As the name Bandits Blend indicates, this is what many believe to be a closest formula to the essential oils likely used by the band of thieves in protecting themselves from the Bubonic Plague. Heralded as the hero that stopped England from the ravage of the Bubonic Plague, King James commuted their death sentence in exchange for the secret of their survival.

The thieves were spice traders who had swept the country, stealing jewellery and possessions from the dead. They revealed to the king they had rubbed essential oils all over their bodies to prevent them from breathing in the fumes of the Black Death. Interestingly, we now know the plague is passed by bites from vermin and in fact were protecting them on a far deeper level.

The recipe for the blend of the "Four Thieves Vinegar" remains in the royal archives today.

1/2 ounce Jojoba oil (or another carrier)

2 drops Clove Bud Essential Oil

3 drops Lemon Essential Oil

2 drops Cinnamon Essential Oil

2 drops Rosemary Essential Oil

1 drop Eucalyptus Essential Oil

Glass Bottle or Container

1. Into a clean glass bottle, add your base carrier oil.

2. Carefully add your essential oils. Place lid on bottle and shake to blend.

3. To use, apply to the bottom of your feet. Another convenient way to use your blend is to carry a pocket diffuser and inhale as you go about your business.

Optional: You may omit the carrier oil to create a synergy blend for diffusing. Diffuse 10-15 minutes in the morning and evening.

Incision and Scar Healing Blend by Marcey DiCaro

4 oz (125ml) Coconut oil (or similar oil Argon is good as is Jojoba))

12 drops Lavender

8 drops Geranium

8 drops Frankincense

5 drops Helichrysm

Make sure the oil is in liquid form - blend well and store in dark brown or blue bottle or jar. Oil may solidify. Apply liberally to scar tissue 1-3 times per day. May use after staples or stitches are removed.

Coconut oil is quite healing for the skin. Lavender, the mother oils is known for it's healing properties for the skin as well as it's soothing the emotions. Geranium is also an excellent skin soother. Frankincense is anti-inflammatory and aids in the healing of wounds as well as internal inflammation. Helichrysm is one of the most healing oils on the earth - it is known for aiding in the healing of bruises, wounds, strains and broken bones. It has great regenerative powers.

Blend for Bruising by Natalie Miller from Aromatic Insights

I used this blend in my practice for:
- 37 year old, female client presenting with bruises to arms, both sides, varying sizes
- Bruising occurred as a result of rough game of roller-skating, roller derby
- She plays as part of a local league on a weekly basis
- Bruising is common as it's a rough and tumble game

A bruise forms when small blood vessels break near the skin's surface, allowing a small amount of blood to leak out under the skin. The trapped blood appears as a black-and-blue mark. As the body reabsorbs the blood with time, the bruise will change colour and eventually disappear.

The aroma blend I recommended to relieve the severity of the bruising comprised the following essential oils:
Origanum marjorana (Sweet Marjoram) – 8 drops
Chamaemelum nobile (Roman Chamomile) – 8 drops
Lavendula officinalis (True Lavender) – 4 drops
Arnica montana (Arnica infused oil) – 20 mls

This formulation makes a 5% blend.

The blend should be lightly massaged into affected areas, soon after the bruises start to appear. Several drops of the blend into the hand, and rubbed into the area lightly should be sufficient for the blend to start working its magic.

Origanum marjorana – has high levels of alcohols which give this oil its warming properties which will help increase blood flow in the area that will allow clearing of the bruise and encouraging cell repair. It also has high monoterpene content which give this oil it analgesic and stimulant properties.
Chamaemelum nobile – has a very high ester content which give this oil its anti-inflammatory properties which would help the bruise and the muscles
Lavendula officinalis – has a high ester content, which give this oil its anti-inflammatory properties, and its high alcohol content give the oil its warming properties
Arnica Montana – has traditionally been used to aid healing of bruises with great reported success

I recommended to the client that the blend be used 2 – 3 times a day on affected area as soon as bruising appears. The bruises starting dissipating within a few days and minimized their severity

Safety Issues:
- *Origanum marjorana* is non-toxic, non-irritant and non-sensitising however most aromatherapy texts suggest it should not be used during pregnancy (hopefully this client wouldn't be playing such a vigorous sport if she were in this condition)
- *Chamaemelum nobile* is considered non-toxic and non-irritant, however Battaglia (1995) reports that contact dermatitis has been reported with topical applications, therefore patch testing should be conducted on people with sensitive skin.
- Although *Lavandula angustifolia* is considered one of the safest essential oils, some people can have allergic reactions to it, and therefore should discontinue use if any allergic reactions occur.

Being Your Own Best Friend Blend – By Julie Nelson of Aromatique Essentials
In a base of organic jojoba oil 25mL

Rose   6 drops

Geranium   3 drops

Jasmine   6 drops

Neroli   6 drops

You can vary the amount of drops so have a play and see what resonates with you!

Or another another blend:

Rose   10 drops

Geranium   3 drops

Jasmine   4 drops

Neroli   6 drops

So many women put their own needs and health to the side and we put our children, partners and family first. It's what we do naturally; we are the nurturers in most cases. We give unconditional love and forget to love ourselves.

We bury our true essence so deeply; we forget how to bring it back. It has been locked away. There can be myriad reasons why we do this as women and it is important for our physical, emotional and spiritual health and wellbeing that we embrace our beautiful essence and allow it to shine beyond our physical bodies.

One divine way to nourish and nurture your beautiful self is by using the above essential oils made up into an anointing perfume. Because these are totally natural ingredients you can use your perfume several times a day. Simply anoint your pulse points, breathe it in and allow the magic of this scent to flow through and beyond you.

Rose otto this amazingly beautiful oil is filled with love and compassion. It is a sensual oil associated to Venus, the Goddess of love and beauty. Besides smelling so beautiful, this oil gives the receiver the essence of beauty and the feminine soul. You will find it is balancing on all levels; it is a supportive and comforting oil indeed.

Geranium is another exquisitely aromatic scent and its key word is balance. Brilliant for balancing your mind, moods and emotions as well as your hormones which, as women, goodness knows...we can do with support in that area at any time in our lives. Geranium is also very nurturing, promoting peace of mind and assists in keeping us grounded in a balanced way for Geranium is another very Venusian oil and associated to Mother Earth.

Jasmine and Neroli are so divinely feminine they give support both emotionally and physically and yes, they are very sensual oils. In fact, like Rose they are considered to have aphrodisiac qualities. Both are balancing. Neroli is quietly strengthening, where Jasmine tends to be more noticed. Jasmine loves to show herself to the world. Both oils are associated to the angelic realm and wrap you up to protect and nurture you when needed.

To bring these beauties together and strengthen their actions I recommend both Vetiver and Patchouli; just a hint of each. They bring mystery, they have a more masculine energy and they give comfort when needed. Patchouli is another aroma classified as an aphrodisiac, where Vetiver helps you to keep your feet planted securely on the ground!

The theme is sensuality, honouring and embracing your feminine essence, in doing so healing begins on other levels and your body, mind connection begins to work in synergy.

You could also add 6 drops of your blend to a bath. Soak it up and breathe it in. Remember it is essential for you to nourish and nurture yourself, give yourself the gift that you so unconditionally give to others.

Conclusion

I would like to say a great big thank you for choosing my book and for sticking with me right to this last page. I hope you have enjoyed it and feel like you have learned a little and thought about a lot. Most of all, I hope you feel you have had value for money!!!! If you think like you would happily have paid for this book, let me ask you, *how much* would you have happily have paid?

Although my name is on the front of this book, it is actually the work of three people (and countless aromatherapists who have gone before) but especially my mum Jill Bruce of The Apothecary and her late husband Michael Cook, who died of pancreatic cancer in January 2010.

An incredible aromatherapist, a dowser of startling ability, and one heck of a chemist, (and possibly the most exasperating man I ever met, incidentally) Michael treated hundreds of thousands of patients, tirelessly travelling the country. If you do feel you would have parted with a few more pennies for this book, I'd love you to give that small amount as a donation to Cancer Research in his name, please. It seems fitting that he will continue to help research that could heal millions of people. Who knows he might even help to fund an essential oil trial that changes the world! I have deliberately kept the price of the book as low as I can in the hope we can achieve this. You can access his donation page through the link on buildyourownreality.com/resources

I'd also ask that if you have found the book useful, please would you leave me a review on Amazon. These really help.

So if you *have* enjoyed it, where do you go now? Well to lesson 2, of course!

The skill of a healer is to see illness as many layers; like an onion, if you like. Peel back one layer and often another lies below. In this book we have done very little more than to look at the onion's brown paper wrapper and half peeled that away. In fact we haven't even given it enough thought to get around to throwing it in the bin!!!

More thought is definitely required if you are going to understand *why* and *how* we get sick.

Illness, particularly recurrent illness, (but not exclusively) often has an underlying cause different from that you might expect.

If you and I went to the supermarket on Friday, and we were both exposed to the same germ ridden air, why have I got a cold on Monday, but you haven't? The body is clearly different in some way, or more specifically, more vulnerable for some reason.

It could be anatomical or physiological; my dodgy lung throws a party at the hint of a chest infection. It likes to show off and opens the door, puts out banners and invites any old low life in. But that might not be the only reason.

Diet is an obvious one, allergies another, even heredity, they can all play a part.

But...

How many of you said...maybe I was run down and stressed?

Good call!

But does that make sense? Could the fact I was fed up with life, lead to me getting ill...?

You bet your bottom dollar it could.

What's more, it usually does, and actually certain illnesses have specific emotions that trigger them too. It's like the body has its own set of linguistic communications, which somehow our generation has forgotten how to hear. In the next book, we look at exactly how this happens and how to interpret the code.

You'll learn how emotions travel from the brain, along electrical impulses and into the tissues of our body. When the mind is fed up, it sends up distress flares through the body.

We uncover the strange mechanisms that not only affect our emotions but even could be causing them too.

We'll delve deep into the physiology of the emotions to find ways to cut the thread that keeps dragging up your same health issues over and over again.

If you are ready to start peeling back more layers of the onion...click here.

Acknowledgments

I am grateful to so many people for their support in the progress of this book. Top of the list is Clare Ella, a remarkable woman who has been an absolute rock at a time when she has been bravely fighting breast cancer. She has tirelessly chivvied, checked and cajoled me. She has read and edited my book between treatments of chemotherapy; her courage and determination seems to know no bounds. She has been an enormous inspiration to me over the past few months and I shall remember both her kindness and conviction for many years to come.

The other therapists involved in the book, Sue Mousley, Annie Day, Erica Strauss, Sharon Falsetto, Dave Jackson, Angela McKay, Rebecca Brink, Julie Nelson, Rebecca Totilo, Marcey DiCaro, and Natalie Miller have transformed this book and I am extremely grateful for both their support but also their confidence and faith in me.

To Mark Bowden, I am always in awe of how commercially astute you are and your boundless energy. My thanks, not only for creating the hypnosis download for my readers, but for being an amazing cheerleader for my cause on days when I needed it most!

Enormous thanks must go to Dr Joann Fletcher and Dr Stephen Buckley of York University Egyptology Department and Dr Lise Manniche of the University of Copenhagen, whose clear and open answers to my questions not only helped to put this book on a much surer footing but revitalised my childhood love for the ancient civilisation and its intriguing culture. The generosity of spirit of sharing so much of your knowledge has moved me a great deal.

The original idea for the book came from Tamara Davison with a long list of ideas for ailments to cover. Her babies Daisy and George seemed to run the risk of reaching adulthood before I finished the ever growing tome, though. Tam, ace idea and thanks so much for giving it to me. Daisy and George, perhaps you might get this book in time to treat your own children!

To Faye, thank you for keeping my feet on the floor and treasured minutes putting the world to rights, climbing the wretched hill! To Helen, my appreciation for cups of tea in far flung cafés and always being willing to entertain my son!

For chocolates, throat tonics, motivational cards in the post, bath oils and as much love as a friend can give, thank you Anna Goodwin. You truly are the friend a girl dreams of and I love you very much for it. For reading, editing, and always being there when I need you both, Liz Thompson and Ariane May. Ariane, here's hoping this book helps you to achieve your dream of helping cancer patients with aromatherapy.

For the most beautiful artwork and a never ending well of patience with me during the cover design process, grateful thanks to Rob of Robert Elsmore Images.

My thanks to my family; to my mum, Jill Bruce, without whom I would have had none of this wisdom to pass on, and to Pat, Neil, Pauline, Richard and Angela for checking up on me.

To my children, none of you ever cease to amaze me. But the largest of my gratitude goes to my lovely husband: I am who I am, because of my history. I *like* who I am because of you. No-one ever gave me a greater gift and one day I hope I can go even half way to repaying you for that.

Directory
Elizabeth Ashley

The Secret Healer

Shropshire, UK

www.thesecrethealer.co.uk

www.buildyourownreality.com

facbook.com/TheSecretHealerWrites

Jill Bruce

Jill Bruce BA (Hons.), LLSA, FECert. is an aromatherapist with many years' experience. She was a founder member of the International Federation of Aromatherapy after having studied at the London School of Aromatherapy. In the 1990's she ran the Jill Bruce School of Aromatherapy which trained hundreds of students to diploma level not only in Aromatherapy, but Anatomy and Physiology, Chemistry and Massage too.

In 1987 she founded *The Apothecary,* which manufactures Clinical Products, Skin Care and Perfume from plants and trades through Etsy.com

She has been a professional astrologer and clairvoyante since 1974, is a member of the Dowsing Research Group and the author of four books, The Garden of Eden, Out of the Labyrinth, The Aura and Wicca Initiation. Last but not least, Jill Bruce is the lady who trained me and the great fortune in life of having given birth to me! Hello Mum!

The Apothecary

Wolverhampton, West Midlands, WV6 8XE, UK

facbook.com/Secret-Knowledge/

www.etsy.com/shop/TheApothecary2

Quote *Secret Healer* at checkout for 20% discounts on blank creams and lotions as well as her skin care and clinical ranges.

Annie Day

Annie runs a successful practice in Staffordshire, England.

Heaven Scent Bliss

Penkridge, Stafford, England. ST19 5LU

www.facbook.com/ComplementaryTherapy

www.heavenscentbliss.co.uk

Quote *Secret Healer* to receive a 10% discount off treatments or training courses.

Clare Ella

Clare Ella runs her aromatherapy practice in Saxilby, Lincoln UK. She graduated from The Tisserand Institute in London in 2000. She sees clients in her clinic and is also building her business to focus on doing home visits to the elderly to help them with fatigue and pain.

Clare Ella Aromatherapy

Saxilby, Lincoln, England. LN1 2PZ

facbook.com/clarellaromatherapy

http://www.clarellaromatherapy.co.uk

Dave Jackson

Ideally Dave will do a face to face consultation in his Cambridge practice, but can do this by phone and or email when face to face when this is not possible.

Cambridge Aromatherapy

Cambridge, England. CB2 9JP

facbook.com/DaveJacksonMassageAndAromatherapy

http://www.cambridgearomatherapy.com

Angie McKay

Angela McKay has been an aromatherapist for over twenty years. After many years working as secondary school psychology teacher, Angie now spends her time writing The Wise Woman's Journal which is available on Amazon.

Wise Woman's Journal

Willenhall, WV13 2RA, UK

facbook.com/Wise-Womans-Journal/

Sue Mousley

Sue is a qualified aromatherapist and trained midwife working in the NHS. She also runs training courses for first aid, aromatherapy in pregnancy and baby massage in her business SOME Training which she runs with business partner, Eunice Owen.

Since Sue still works part time in the NHS, places on her courses are limited so therefore we are not offering a blanket discount. However, please quote *Secret Healer* at booking and discrete conversations about possible discounts can begin!!!

SOME Training Ltd

Nuneaton. Warwickshire, CV10 7GG

www.sometrainingltd.co.uk

Recommended Training School

The Institute of Traditional Herbal Medicine & Aromatherapy (ITHMA)

Principal: Gabriel Mojay LicAc,CertEd,FIFPA

Courses held at Regent's University, Regent's Park, London NW1

Tel: 020 7193 7383

info@aromatherapy-studies.com

http://www.aromatherapy-studies.com

Mark Bowden Hypnotherapy

Mark is the creator of the free relaxation hypnosis download that comes with this book. He runs a successful hypnotherapy practice and a thriving online store of his recorded downloads on Amazon.

Plymouth, Devon, UK

facbook.com/mbhypno

www.markbowdenhypnotherapy.co.uk

Marks free relaxation download is available at buildyourownreality.com/free-hypnosis-download/

US Therapists

Rebecca Brink

Rebeccas practice involves gently stretching your body while you relax into and deepen your range of motion. Trigger point therapy is an important element of her work with the patient to help relieve muscle tension, aches and pains and to help bring the body into a healthier state. She uses essential oils to enhance the experience and help bring added relief to chronic problem areas of the body. She feels that with regular yoga practice, thai bodywork and essential oils you can bring your body back to a place of health and homeostasis.

Serenity Thai Bodywork

serenitybodywork7@gmail.com

Marcey DiCaro

Marcey DiCaro holds a Masters Degree in counselling, psychology, hypnotherapy, quantum lightweaving healing and is a certified aromatherapist.

She began working with essential oils 30 years ago and in the past 10 years she met and studied with her mentor, Mikael Zayat a 3rd generation alchemist from Quebec. From him she not only learned the science of the oils, but also the energetic connection with the oils. Her favorite study was spending a day with a grove of trees and noting their interactions with their surrounding and the energies they transmitted.

She is passionate about her healing work and sees essential oils as one of the tools she employs, to assist people in connecting with their inner wisdom and truth. From that place, healing occurs.

The Essential Alchemist

Tucson, AZ. 85742 United States

1-520-490-4149

Please quote *Secret Healer* for a 10% discount on treatments given by Marcey.

Sharon Falsetto

Sharon is a UK-certified aromatherapist with over seven years experience of living and working in the United States as an aromatherapist. She is the author of the book *Authentic Aromatherapy*. Sharon founded the business *Sedona Aromatherapie* in 2007, a home study aromatherapy school, custom aromatherapy blending service for therapists, spas, hotels and more, and offers a full range of writing and editing services to the aromatherapy industry. Sharon is the Arizona Regional Director, past Board member, and current co-editor of the Journal for the *National Association for Holistic Aromatherapy* (NAHA). She lives in Sedona, Arizona.

Sedona Aromatherapy

Sedona, Arizona, USA

facbook.com/SedonaAromatherapy

www.sedonaaromatherapie.com

Please quote Secret Healer at checkout for a 5% discount.

Erica Straus

Healing Essence

Oakland, CA 94606 United States

Erica first became interested in aromatherapy when it helped her to get off of some of the many painkillers that she took for everything from headaches to backaches. She was very ill at the time and impressed with the power of essential oils. She decided to study aromatherapy in order to help herself to heal. During her study she discovered a passion for both aromatherapy and massage.

She was living in London at the time and began offering aromatherapy massage to others. She then returned to California (after 20 years abroad) and in order to become certified to perform massage in the state, was required to accumulate hours at a California massage school. This instigated a new journey of bodywork discovery, adding more modalities and specialist knowledge to her expertise. She is now an instructor at a massage school in Oakland, California, however she says "I doubt that my personal journey of bodywork education will ever end (because there is always more to learn!)".

In 2011, her friends and family persuaded her to sell some of the blends she was making for them and her business, Healing Essence was born. She feels very strongly about only using organic essential oils and base oils, and created a small line of 100% organic aromatherapy products, which she hand-blends. In her massage practice she uses only use organic massage oils.

Her most common mix contains arnica and essential oils that are anti-inflammatory, muscle relaxing and pain relieving. She can, as an alternative, custom blend massage oils or personal roll-ons for specific conditions and symptoms.

She does house calls around San Francisco and the East Bay. She offers massage in a number of modalities, with or without organic aromatherapy oils. Her work frequently integrates Swedish, Deep Tissue, Sports Massage and Shiatsu. In addition she offers more specialized massages such as Lymphatic Drainage, Prenatal and Postnatal Massage, and has experience in working with chronic diseases and disabilities. Her work combines scientific knowledge with an intuitive approach for a truly outstanding and effective experience. She also offers a range of hand-blended organic aromatherapy products through her Healing Essence online shop and local retailers.

www.healing-essence-massage.com

www.healingessenceshop.com

Rebecca Totilo

Tampa Bay, US

Rebecca's flair and passion for life bursts into living color when she writes and speaks, and you can see in the visual way she presents herself. She believes very strongly in the "show, don't tell" principle in everything she does. She has ministered to literally millions of people via television, radio and live appearances.

She is an award-winning published author of over 40 books, including: Through the Night With God, The Official Christian Babysitting Guide, The Christian Girls Guide to Money, and His Majesty Requests. Her credits include working as a contributor writer on two best-selling series (Quiet Moments with God and Stories for the Teens Heart) which sold over one million and five million copies respectively. She is also a freelance writer for several national magazines include Christian Parenting Today, Discipleship Journal and Womans World.

Rebeccas photography work has appeared in numerous national magazines such as Womans World, Sports Spectrum, Evangel, and Sharing the Victory. But by far, her greatest accomplishment, if you asked her, is after a decade of rejection slips (with almost 150 in one year!), Rebecca hit it big in 1999, with over 13 books contracts, ranging from teaching curriculum to gift books and devotionals for adults. Truly, its her grit determination that makes her inspirational writings draw such a mass market appeal.

Rebecca graduated from Virginia Commonwealth University in 1986 with a Bachelors of Science Degree in Information Systems. In addition, she attended Faith Bible Institute in Richmond, Virginia for instruction in ministry and University of the Nations (Youth With A Mission) Discipleship Training and Basic Leadership Schools. She served in missions with YWAMs Kings Kids and Teen Challenge.

Rebecca has been a homeschool mom for 21 years. In addition to all this, she is the president and publisher of Rebecca at the Well Foundation, a Judeo-Christian international organization which publishes literary works that prepare the Bride for the Messiahs return. For over a decade now, Rebecca has been teaching believers about the Hebrew roots of the faith on an international basis.

Rebecca owns a cute soap boutique, Aroma Hut, near the beach where she practices as an aromatherapist. She offers online courses on aromatherapy and perfume making . She specializes in educating people on essential oils from a biblical prospective. Her understanding of Scriptures richly woven with the tapestry of the ancient Hebrew customs makes her inspirational works truly memorable.

Aroma Hut Institute offers professional quality clinical aromatherapy courses online and in-person. Aroma Hut training includes Aromatherapy Certification programs for Level 1 Foundation (50 hours) & Level 2 Advanced Clinical (200 hours).

Courses are approved for Massage Therapy CEU's in Florida and Nationally through NCBTMB and can be taken individually. Graduates have the option to continue with Teacher Training and start their own Aroma Hut School.

She is a best-selling author of over 40 books on aromatherapy and essential oils including, Organic Beauty With Essential Oil, Therapeutic Blending With Essential Oil and Heal With Oil. She has been seen by millions via national television, syndicated radio, and internet.She has over twenty-five years of experience as an international educator, specializing in the ancient biblical healing arts.

www.healwithoil.com

facbook.com/rebecca.totilo

Australia

Natalie Miller

Natalie's aromatherapy qualifications are relatively new, but her aromatic journey began many years ago. During her mid 20's, she had become interested in holistic healing when she suffered a very deep depression. She looked at aromatherapy, crystals and meditation, but never really took them that seriously. Fifteen years later things began to change for her.
This is what she has to say....

"In my early 40's, after falling into another depression pit, I came across a two books which changed my view of the world – "You Sexy Mother" (by Jodie Hedley-Ward) and "Like Chocolate for Women" (by Kim Morrison and Fleur Whelligan). Inspired by these books, I decided to write a "Living Life List" aka a bucket list. One of the many things on the list was to learn aromatherapy.

Armed with this inspiration, I enrolled in a two year Diploma of Aromatherapy course (nothing like jumping in the deep end). At the successful completion of my course, I started my business, combining my past experiences in the adult education, training and coaching arena with my aromatherapy knowledge. Aromatic Insights was born.

An avid social media user, I have connected with aromatherapists around the world, regularly contributing to various groups, sites and pages in the never ending endeavour to learn more, to improve myself and grow. I am a full member of the Australian aromatherapy association, IAAMA, and run a Facbook group for Australian aromatherapists called "Australian Aromatherapy."

Aromatic Insights,

Melbourne, Australia

aromaticinsights@hotmail.com

facbook.com/AromaticInsights

Quote Secret Healer for a 5% discount on treatments.

Julie Nelson

Diploma in Aromatherapy & Certificate IV in Natural Beauty Certificare IV in Workplace Training and Assessment

Certificate III in Astrology

Certificate in Bach Flowers

This is what Julie has to say about her business:

Your scent is as unique as your fingerprint. This is why I create exquisite products perfectly aligned to your distinct essence.

I believe in the Sacred Primal. This means, as a Holistic Aromatherapist, I am guided by instinctual as well as medicinal knowledge. With almost 20 years professional experience, **as a practitioner, educator and c**onsultant, I am highly regarded as a formidable authority in my field.

I believe true beauty resides in your soul. Cultivating beauty is, to me, the essential sacrament of self-care.

Aromatique Essentials are the highest quality, bespoke skin-food and soul-crafted perfumes individually tailored to your precise needs.

My integrity demands that Aromatique Essentials uses **truly organic and truly natural essential oils.**

I fell in love with essential oils and the art of aromatherapy around the time I fell in love with my newborn baby girl. The nose knows who we love and what we are meant to do.

My beautiful daughter was born with many complications and challenges. She was the youngest and smallest TOF (tracheoesophageal fistula) baby born in Australia at that time.

As a mother I desperately wanted to do more for her and support her in every way possible. Using aromatherapy on a daily basis improved her early life and transformed us physically, emotionally and spiritually.

Filled with deep gratitude for this gift from Nature, I devoted my life to learning how aromatherapy can support and enhance the well-being of others.

Today I have almost 20 years experience as Holistic Practitioner, Aromatherapy Consultant and Aromatherapy Coach. Having 13 years experience as a professional educator I was responsible for the design and delivery of Aromatherapy and Beauty programs for Australia's leading natural therapies colleges.

My expertise has been featured in national publications like Pharmacy Trade, Pregnancy Magazine, Cleo, For Me, Body & Soul, Good Weekend, Sydney Morning Herald as well as health and beauty blogs and radio segments.

But essentially, I am an alchemist, healer and teacher. It is my divine calling. And I warmly invite you to experience the gift of my sacred mission.

My deepest wish is for you to experience the profound healing, vitality and sensual abundance that aromatherapy has blessed my life with.

Discover your divine essence. Let me enhance the scent of your soul.

Aromatique Essentials Artisan Perfume Workshop

Learn how to design and create your 'Signature Scent' with my guidance with the use of my personal collection of essential oils containing some gorgeous exotiques that are not available to the public!

- Do you love wearing perfume but you cannot wear commercial perfumes?
- Would you like to expand your knowledge and discover the world of true natural perfumery?
- Then this artisan perfume workshop is for YOU!

Indulge in the mystique of traditional artisan perfume making & discover the extraordinary and beautiful world of natural perfumery -

What the day involves

- On arrival meet and greet whilst enjoying a range of boutique teas and a delicious high tea including decadent vegan sweets.

- Introduction to perfume blending, covering the basic principles of blending to create your own signature scent

- Identify your personal and favourite essential oil aromas

- Learn the difference between natural chemicals versus synthesised chemicals

- Enjoy the experience of creating one-of-a kind perfume, I will guide you every step of the way

- A handcrafted pendant is gifted to you to decorate your bottle (made from costume jewellery from the 1920s-1960s, there are no two the same

- Your perfume can be in a base of rose or orange blossom floral water size 50ml as a perfume spray, OR choose organic jojoba as the base, size 25ml as an anointing perfume

- We close the day with a glass of champagne as you celebrate *'Capturing the Essence of You' in your unique signature perfume.*

Connect and Embrace with Your Beautiful Essence

My passion for perfumes has always existed. Wearing perfume to me is a ritual to honour my feminine self, but it is much more than that.

A quote from Helen Keller best describes the power of scent…

"Smell is the potent wizard that transports you across thousands of miles and all the years you have lived"

How true it is! When working with beautiful natural scents I am often taken on a journey back in time and I find myself smiling, sometimes chuckling, other times teary as my mind fills with beautiful and happy memories.

Wearing your own signature perfume brings balance in to your day, uplifts your emotions, reduces stress, anxiety and depression. All it takes is one breath in and you are wrapped in an unquestionable veil of euphoria.

Your body and mind begin to relax and let go, you realise you are wearing a smile, your breathing becomes more rhythmic...

For myself, I feel lighter emotionally. Whenever I breathe in any one of my signature perfumes I release a sigh with a smile and experience pure bliss

A note from Julie:

This workshop has been created with the greatest intentions, filled with my passion and love to help bring you more confidence, sel-love and self-empowerment into your beautiful life.

My wish is that you embrace and connect with the essence of who you are through the daily ritual of applying your signature scent.

Aromatique Essentials

Blackheath, NSW, Australia

facbook.com/aromatiqueessentials

www.aromatiqueessentials.com.au

Quote Secret Healer for a 10% discount on products and courses. Spend over $100 and receive a free vial of the perfume of your choice.

Taiwan

Richard Yu - Contact for Hinoki Essential Oil

5% discount on regular prices when the reader quotes *Secret Healer*

Presently - prices are as follows. (before discount)

10 ml   - USD$ 14.80

30 ml   - USD$ 38.80

50 ml   - USD$ 58.00

Wholesale quantity negotiable price - minimum 25 kg or 25000 ml.

price exclude shipping cost - additional price if large order (sample 10 ml / 30 ml free shipping) - usually by airmail (unless package too large by air)

Aquagreen Co Ltd

2F-6, NO.137-1 FU SHUN RD HSI-TUN DIST. , TAI-CHUNG, TAIWAN

Tel: 886-4-2463-5527

Fax: 886-4-2463-6053

aqua.green@msa.hinet.net

aquagreencomtw@gmail.com

www.aquagreen.com.tw

Medical Glossary

Adapted from essentialoils.co.za/glossary.htm

Absolute The most concentrated form of fragrance obtained when distilling a concrete

Allergy Hypersensitivity caused by a foreign substance

Alopecia Baldness – can be temporary or permanent

Amenorrhoea The absence of menstruation

Anaerobic Type of organism that does not require oxygen

Analgesic Relieving or deadening pain

Anaphrodisiac Lessening sexual desire

Anemia Deficiency of either quantity or quality of red corpuscles in the blood

Anesthetic Pain relieving by loss of sensation

Anti-acid Combats acid in the body

Anti-arthritic An agent which helps to combat arthritis

Anti-allergenic Reduces symptoms of allergies

Antibacterial Fights bacterial growth

Antibiotic   Fights infection in the body by preventing the growth or destroying bacteria

Anti-convulsant   Helps control convulsions

Anti-depressant   Helps to counteract depression and lifts the mood

Anti-emetic   Reduces the severity or incidence of vomiting

Anti-fungal   Prevents the growth of fungi

Anti-galactagogue   Impedes or lessens the flow of milk

Anti-hemorrhagic   A substance preventing or combating bleeding

Antihistamine   Counteracts allergic reaction

Anti-infectious   Prevents against infection

Anti-microbial   A substance reducing or resisting microbes

Antioxidant   A substance to prevent or delay oxidation

Anti-parasitic   Acts against parasites

Anti-phlogistic   Counteracts inflammation

Anti-pruritic   Relieves or prevents sensation of itching

Anti-pyretic   Reduces fever

Anti-rheumatic   An agent which helps to combat rheumatism

Anti-sclerotic   Helps to prevent hardening of arteries

Anti-seborrheic   Helps control the oily secretion from sweat glands

Antiseptic   A substance helping to control infection

Anti-spasmodic   A substance to help prevent and ease spasms and relieve cramps

Anti-sudorific   A substance to help lessen sweating

Anti-toxic   Antidote or treatment to counteract the effects of poison

Anti-tussive   Relieves coughing

Aphrodisiac   Increasing sexual desire and sexual functioning

Aromatherapy   The therapeutic use of essential oils

Arrhythmia   Irregular or loss of heartbeat rhythm

Arteriosclerosis   Hardening of the arteries

Astringent   Causing contraction of organic tissue

Atherosclerosis   Accumulation of fatty deposits on the inside walls of arteries

Atony   Lack of muscle tone

Bactericidal   An agent destroying bacteria

Balsam   Water soluble, semi-solid or viscous resinous exudate similar to that of gum

Balsamic   Soothing medicine or application having the qualities of balsam

Bechic   Anything referring to coughing, or an agent relieving cough

Biennial   A plant completing its life cycle in two years, without flowering the first year

Bilious   A condition caused by an excessive secretion of bile

Blepharitis   Inflammation of the eyelids

Calmative   A sedative

Carcinogenic   A substance that promotes cancer or cancerous growths

Cardiac   Pertaining to the heart

Carminative   Settles the digestive system and relieves flatulence

Carrier oil   An oil which is used to dilute essential oils for the purpose of massage - see fixed oils

Cellulite   An "orange peel" effect caused by local accumulation of fat and waste products

Cephalic   A substance stimulating and clearing the mind

Glossary of essential oil terms essential oil words terms explained

Chemotypes   The same botanical species occurring in other forms due to different growth conditions

Chi / Qi   Chinese term referring to the essential life force

Cholagogue   Stimulating the secretion of bile into the duodenum

Cholecystokenetic   Agent that stimulates the contraction of the gall bladder

Choleretic   Helps the liver to excrete bile, leading to greater bile flow

Cholesterol   Is a steroid alcohol found in red blood cells, bile, nervous tissue and animal fat

Cicatrisation Formation of scar tissue

Cicatrisant   Agent promoting healing by scar tissue formation

Cirrhosis   Chronic inflammation and degeneration of any organ (normally in the liver)

Clinical trial A controlled study to look at the effectiveness of a specific ingredient or application

Cohobation   Is a process in the extraction method of especially rose essential oil, to ensure a "complete" oil

Cold pressed Refers to a method of extraction where no external heat is applied during the process

Colic Pain due to contraction of the muscle of the abdominal organs

Colitis Inflammation of the colon

Concrete   A waxy concentrate semi-solid essential oil extract, made from plant material, and is used to make an absolute

Constipation A state where normal bowel functions are not present

Cystitis Bladder inflammation

Cytophylactic Action of increasing the leukocyte activity to defend the body against infection

Cytotoxic Toxic to all cells

Decoction A herbal preparation made by boiling the material and reducing it to a concentration

Decongestant A substance which helps to relieve congestion

Demulcent An agent protecting mucus membranes and helps stop irritation

Depurative Helps to detoxify and to combat impurities in the blood and body

Dermatitis Inflammation of the skin

Detoxifier Helps to detoxify and to combat impurities in the blood and body

Diaphoretic A substance which helps to promote perspiration

Diffuser A device which helps to release the fragrance molecules into the air

Distillation   A method of extraction used in the manufacture of essential oils

Diuretic   Helps to produce urine and remove water from the body

Dysmenorrhoea   Painful menstruation

Emmenagogue   Inducing or assisting menstruation

Emollient   Softening and soothing to the skin

Emphysema   Degenerative disease of the lungs where the air sacs become enlarged

Endocrine   Pertaining to the ductless glands

Essential oil   Volatile aromatic liquid constituting the odorous principles of botanical matter

Expectorant   A substance that helps to expel mucus from the lungs

Expression   Is an extraction method where essential oils are pressed to obtain the oil

Febrifuge   Helps to combat fever

Fibrillation   Rapid twitching of muscle fiber

Flower water The water resulting from the distillation of essential oils, which still contains some of the properties of the plant material used in the extraction

Fold Refers to the percentage of terpenes removed by re-distillation - single fold to fivefold

Fractionated oils Refers to oils that have been re-distilled, either to have terpenes removed or to remove other substances

Fungicide A substance which destroys fungal infections

Gingivitis Inflammation of the gums

Glossitis Inflammation of the tongue

Halitosis Bad breath

Hematuria / Haematuria Presence of blood in the urine

Hemorrhoids Piles which are dilated rectal veins

Hemostatic Helps to stop bleeding

Hepatic Pertaining to the liver

Hepatoxic An agent having a toxic or harmful effect on the liver

Herpes Inflammation of the skin or mucus membranes

Hormone   A product from living cells that produces a specific activity of cells remote from its point of origin

Hybrid   A plant created by fertilization of one species by another

Hydrodiffusion   Is a distillation method of essential oil extraction where the steam is produced above the botanical material and then percolates down

Hydrosol   Floral water

Hyperglycemia / Hyperglycaemia Excess of sugar in the blood

Hypertension   High blood pressure

Hypocholesterolemia   Lowering of the cholesterol content of the blood

Hypoglycemia   Lowered blood sugar levels

Hypotension Abnormally low blood pressure

Infused oil   An oil produced by steeping the macerated botanical material in oil until the oil has taken on some of the material's properties

Infusion   Herbal remedy made by steeping the plant material in water

Laxative   A substance that helps with bowel movements

Macerate   To soak until soft

Massage therapist   A person qualified to perform therapeutic massage on people

Massage therapy   The manipulation of soft tissue to enhance health and general well-being

Menopause   The normal cessation of menstruation

Mucolytic   Breaking down mucus

Myelin cells   Fatty material enveloping the majority of nerve

Narcotic   Substance inducing sleep

Nephritis   Inflammation of the kidneys

Nervine   Substance that strengthens and tones the nerves and nervous system

Neuralgia   Stabbing pain along a nerve pathway

Neurotoxin   A substance having a toxic or harmful effect on the nervous system

Oedema   Water retention

Oleo gum resin   Odoriferous exudation from botanical material consisting of essential oil, gum and resin

Oleoresin   Natural resinous exudation from plants or aromatic liquid preparation extracted from botanical material

Olfaction   Sense of smell

Olfactory bulb   The center where the processing of smell is started and is then passed onto other areas of the brain

Oxidation   Related to the addition of oxygen to an organic molecule, or the removal of electrons or hydrogen from the molecule

Palpitations Undue awareness of heartbeat, or rapid heartbeat or abnormal rhythm of the heart

Pathogenic   An agent causing or producing disease

Peptic Pertaining to gastric secretions as well as areas affected by them

Perennial   A plant living for more than two years

Prophylactic Preventative of disease or infection

Prostatitis   Inflammation of the prostate gland

Pruritis   Itching

Psoriasis   A chronic skin disease characterized by red patches and silver scaling

Psychosomatic   Pertaining to the mind and body

Pulmonary   Pertaining to the lungs

Rectification   Process of re-distilling essential oils to rid them of certain constituents

Renal   Pertaining to the kidneys

Resin   Natural or prepared product - natural resins are exudations from trees, prepared resins are oleoresins from which the essential oil has been removed

Resinoids   Perfumed material extracted from natural resinous material by solvent extraction

Rubefacient   Substance causing redness and possible irritation to the skin

Sciatica   Pain down the back of the legs in the area serviced by the sciatic nerve

Sclerosis   Hardening of tissue due to inflammation

Seborrhea   Increased secretion of sebum

Sialogogue   An agent stimulating the secretion of saliva

Soporific   A substance which helps to induce sleep

Stomachic   A substance which helps with the digestion and helps to improve appetite

Stomatitis   Inflammation of the mucus membranes of the mouth

Styptic   An agent that stops external bleeding

Sudorific   An agent causing sweating

Synergy   Agents working together and in harmony to produce an effect greater than the sum of the two separate agents

Tachycardia Abnormally increased heartbeat

Thrombosis   The formation of a blood clot

Thrush   A fungal infection in the mouth or vaginal area

Tic   Repetitive twitching

Tincture   Referring to either a herbal or perfume material prepared in an alcohol base

Glossary of essential oil terms essential oil words terms explained

Unguent   A soothing or healing salve or balm

Urticaria   Weal on the skin

Vasoconstrictor   An agent causing the contraction of blood vessel walls

Vasodilator   An agent causing the dilation of blood vessel walls

Vermifuge   An agent expelling intestinal worms

Volatile   Substance that is unstable and evaporates easily, like an essential oil

Vulnerary   An agent applied externally which helps to heal wounds and sores and helps to prevent tissue degeneration

About the Author

Elizabeth Ashley qualified as an aromatherapist in 1993, and then passed her Advanced Aromatherapy Diploma in 1994. She has been practicing aromatherapy for almost 21 years.

In 1999, she fell into a whole new career in the aggressive commercial sector of recruitment consultancy. There she discovered her father's second hand car salesman genes had passed along and found she had quite a gift of the gab! More than that, she discovered she could sell...and then some.

In 2008, Elizabeth fell ill during pregnancy with a blood clot in her lungs. The pulmonary embolism prevented her from working and she started to write. Very quickly she gained her first contract as a ghost writer...a recipe book for cheese cakes!

In 2010 she was published professionally for her work on Galbanum oil in the Aromatherapy Thymes, journal of the International Federation of Aromatherapists, and on Tuberose oil by the New Zealand Register of Holistic Therapist.

In 2011 she was seconded on a consultative basis to Walsall Independent Treatment Centre, designed to be a rainbow bridge between traditional and complementary medicines. There she became aware of the rumblings of change in healthcare. Her book *Sales Strategies for Gentle Souls* explains the connotations of this.

Many of her books are aimed at helping qualified aromatherapists to expand their healing repertoire and build their businesses. She also writes for people who have an interest in essential oils and want to learn how to heal. Her in depth essential oil profiles chart the healing properties of plants from the most arcane depths of historic folklore up to the scientific lab trials of today.

In 2014 she ranks in the top 50 contract writers on the freelancer marketplace Elance.com. She is the ghost writer of seven number one Amazon best sellers in the natural healing category. She lives in Shropshire with her husband and youngest son, kept company by their cat, the budgie and many shoals of tropical fish! Her elder son and daughter attend University and make her prouder than anything ever could.

Elizabeth Ashley is possibly one of the most published aromatherapy writers you have never heard of! By 2015, all of that will have changed. Elizabeth Ashley is *The Secret Healer*.

Other books in The Secret Healer Series
Available on Amazon from 30.11.14

Book 2 Essential Oils for Mind Body Spirit
The Holistic Medicine of Clinical Aromatherapy

Healing the skin, easing the tummy ache or getting someone to sleep is easy with essential oils. Anyone can do it. The joy of healing, though, comes from peeling back the layers of the disease, almost like a detective to find out exactly what caused it in the first place.

Consider this book to be lesson 2 in The Secret Healer Series.

You have mastered which oil to use for what and why...this book takes you step by step though the ancient healing mechanisms of the aura, the chakras and meridians but also explores how that ties in with the latest scientific discoveries into how the emotions affect our health. Using Candace Pert's remarkable "Molecules of Emotion" research, The Secret Healer shows you *where* to look for healing links and *why*.

- Uncover how a certain recurrent negative emotion can be the trigger to make you ill?

- Understand internal processes that mean that psychology, neurology and immunology are quintessentially, and inextricably linked.
- Learn how to use essential oils control your emotions and in turn bring about a far greater standard of wellness.
- Discover mindblowing research that shows the emotions we experience are actually the sensations of neuropeptides triggering our organs to do their jobs
- Reflect on the wonder of Chinese medicine and ancient healing being completely accurate in their healing mechanisms for thousands of years...now that science proves it to be so.

Essential Oils for The Mind Body Spirit couples ancient wisdom with cutting edge science. This is the knowledge the drug companies hope you never find out and our doctors pray we all will.

A short write up, for a book that will change your life. I promise you, when you read the latest findings of psychoimmunolgy, you will never waster another day on being angry again.

Book 3 The Essential Oil Liver Cleanse

The Professional Aromatherapist's Liver Detox

We are warned of the threats of heart attacks, strokes and cancer, especially if we are overweight.

What is kept quieter is doctors have established a link between toxicity in the liver and metabolic syndrome, the condition that leads to many of these conditions. What's more non fatty liver disease is known to underlie many other conditions such as ezcema, allergies and headaches.

The scandal is just how many of our livers are struggling under the strain of over processed foods, pharmaceutical debris and actually even our own bad tempers!

This book explains:

- The importance of the liver and its functions
- How it becomes dysfunctional and how to interpret warning signposts
- How to cleanse and nourish using not just essential oils, but also vitamins and minerals and diet.
- The strange correlation between how our emotions translate negativity into disease.

- How to implement other therapies such as chiropractic, acupressure and counselling and how to secure fantastic referrals.

This book is best used in tandem with The Professional Stress Solution to benefit from the complementary healing. Use Sales Strategies for Gentle Souls to create a marketing plan to use your new found knowledge to smash your competition out of the water!!!

Book 4 The Professional Stress Solution
Essential Oils and Holistic Health Stress Management Techniques for The Professional Aromatherapist

Stress is pandemic in our society.

Scientists agree it plays a quintessential role in how likely it is we will suffer from chronic and possibly fatal illnesses in the future. Risk factors of metabolic syndrome, diabetes, stroke and heart disease are increased through stress.

The daft thing is....aromatherapy can do amazing things to ease it, and potentially aromatherapists could take a massive workload away from the doctor's surgeries.

- Discover the hormonal changes and peptide triggers that change a person's health and mental state.
- Learn how it affects the liver, adrenals and pituitary gland.
- Uncover the strange phenomenon of Yin disease
- Build a better foundation of care, but also a knowledge base that means you can sell your treatments more effectively.
- Improve your healing skills set
- Supercharge your referrals potential from other complementary therapists and orthodox medicine alike.

Includes free bonus material of

- Chiropractic chart of misalignments and potential organic disturbance
- Chart of the meridians and suggested acupressure points to detox the organs more quickly
- Detailed information about how to improve the patients condition with vitamin and minerals therapy
- In depth dietary advice
- Free hypnotherapy relaxation download

Essential Oils are The Off Switch for stress. The *Professional Stress Solution* is the ON SWITCH for your aromatherapy business.

Book 5 The Aromatherapy Eczema Treatment
Healing Eczema, Itchy Skin Rashes and Atopic Dermatitis with Essential Oils and Holistic Medicine

Most people appreciate that the itching and redness of eczema can be used using essential oils, but what if I told you they were capable of so much more?

Imagine if, as a therapist, you were able to pinpoint the emotions that set off these flares? Can you visualise what it would mean to your patient if you were able to isolate the very protagonist causing the eczema breakout and alleviate their pain completely?

Well now you can.

This book teaches you:

- How to isolate the emotions causing the emotional cycle of pain

- The likely food triggers for your patient and the tools to identify the exact times they will detonate a reaction
- The familial traits and links that lead to atopic eczema
- How these links connect with the liver and in turn how to cleanse the liver toxicity
- Vitamins and minerals to cleanse and nourish the system

The book contains very real that will not only transform the way you treat clients, but will skyrocket your clinic's takings.

I recommend reading this book in tandem with *The Professional Stress Solution* and the *Essential Oil Liver Cleanse* to fully understand the cycles and processes of treatment. Add to it *Sales Strategies for Gentle Souls* and your business will stand on an entirely new footing.

Sales Strategies for Gentle Souls
Targeted Sales Training for Professional Aromatherapists

Wonderful things are happening in complementary therapy. Very gifted people are churning out fantastic research and results. The internet is full of what essential oils can do. But when a gentle soul emerges from their relaxing haze of their aromatherapy class room, how do they harness the buzz of energy around them for their craft?

From 1999-2008 I worked in one of the most aggressive commercial environments there is. My role as a recruitment consultant was 80% cold calling in am extremely saturated sales arena. Despite my own gentle soul, I found ways not only to compete, but to excel.

- Learn how to pinpoint the best customers for your practice
- Cost your treatments to ensure every treatment is profitable for both you and your customer
- Discover how to make every conversation into a potential sale lead without becoming a complete and utter pain in the a*s!
- Uncover the reasons why you are not closing sales so you never have to make the same mistakes again
- Create a growth environment where you plan success and always find yourself stepping into it

If you are working with essential oils, and you want to make a good living for it, then you need to learn to sell. What's more, if you are going to say "selling doesn't work on my customers"....then you have simply been taught to do it wrongly.

My dream is to see aromatherapy at the forefront of medicine. I need an army of gifted healers to achieve that. Consider yourself to be my newest recruit and I am going to drill you till you are the slickest, subtlest and most effective marketeer there is. You have the knowledge to make people better, now let me give you the business prowess to heal even more people than you have ever done before.

The Secret Healer has stress in her sights and she's about to make a killing. Listen carefully...she has much to tell you. £1.99 / $2.99

www.thesecrethealer.co.uk

www.buildyourownreality.com

In 2015, Elizabeth Ashley will also publish a new essential oil profile on Amazon each week. See her author profile on Amazon for the latest releases.

Works Cited

Amsterdam JD1, S. J. (2012, 10 18). *Chamomile (Matricaria recutita) may provide antidepressant activity in anxious, depressed humans: an exploratory study.* Retrieved 10 18, 2014, from Pubmed: http://www.ncbi.nlm.nih.gov/pubmed/22894890

Asadi-Shahmirzadi A1, M. S.-E. (2012, 12 21). *Benefit of Aloe vera and Matricaria recutita mixture in rat irritable bowel syndrome: Combination of antioxidant and spasmolytic effects.* Retrieved 10 18, 2014, from Pubmed: http://www.ncbi.nlm.nih.gov/pubmed/23263994

Ben Slima A, A. M. (2013, 03 07). *Antioxidant properties of Pelargonium graveolens L'Her essential oil on the reproductive damage induced by deltamethrin in mice as compared to alpha-tocopherol.* Retrieved 10 18, 2014, from Pubmed: http://www.ncbi.nlm.nih.gov/pubmed/23496944

Bigos M1, W. M. (2012, 08 28). *Antimicrobial activity of geranium oil against clinical strains of Staphylococcus aureus.* Retrieved 10 18, 2014, from Pubmed: http://www.ncbi.nlm.nih.gov/pubmed/22929626

Boukhris M1, B. M. (2012, 06 26). *Hypoglycemic and antioxidant effects of leaf essential oil of Pelargonium graveolens L'Hér. in alloxan induced diabetic rats*. Retrieved 10 18, 2014, from Pubmed: http://www.ncbi.nlm.nih.gov/pubmed/22734822

Bozzuto G1, C. M. (2011, 01). *Tea tree oil might combat melanoma*. Retrieved 10 18, 2014, from Pubmed: http://www.ncbi.nlm.nih.gov/pubmed/20560116

Bruce, J. (1994). Advanced Diploma of Aromatherapy. *Jill Bruce School of Aromatherapy* .

Bruce, J. (1993). Diploma Course of Aromatherapy. *Jill Bruce School of Aromatherapy* .

Bruce, J. (1993). *The Garden of Eden* . Walsall: Magdalena Press.

Cemek M1, K. S. (2008, 06). *Antihyperglycemic and antioxidative potential of Matricaria chamomilla L. in streptozotocin-induced diabetic rats*. Retrieved 10 18, 2014, from http://www.ncbi.nlm.nih.gov/pubmed/18404309

Chandrashekhar VM1, H. K. (2012, 09 01). *Anti-allergic activity of German chamomile (Matricaria recutita L.) in mast cell mediated allergy model*. Retrieved 10 18, 2014, from Pubmed: http://www.ncbi.nlm.nih.gov/pubmed/21651969

Chin KB1, C. B. (2013, 12 12). *The effect of tea tree oil (Melaleuca alternifolia) on wound healing using a dressing model.* Retrieved 10 18, 2014, from Pubmed: http://www.ncbi.nlm.nih.gov/pubmed/23848210

Davis, P. (1993). *Aromatherapy and A-Z.* Saffron Waldron, Essex: C W Daniel Company.

Di Campli E1, D. B. (2012, 11). *Activity of tea tree oil and nerolidol alone or in combination against Pediculus capitis (head lice) and its eggs.* Retrieved 10 18, 2014, from Pubmed: http://www.ncbi.nlm.nih.gov/pubmed/22847279

Dolati K, R. H. (2013). *Effect of aqueous fraction of Rosa damascena on ileum contractile response of guinea pigs.* Retrieved 10 11, 2014, from Pubmed: http://www.ncbi.nlm.nih.gov/pubmed/25050281

Effects of plant extracts on the reversal of glucose-induced impairment of stress-resistance in Caenorhabditis elegans. (2014, 03). Retrieved 10 18, 2014, from Pubmed: http://www.ncbi.nlm.nih.gov/pubmed/24390728

El-Sayed S. Abdel-Hameed, 1. ,. (2013, 27 10). *Characterization of the Phytochemical Constituents of Taif Rose and Its Antioxidant and Anticancer Activities.* Retrieved 10 12, 2014, from Pubmed: http://www.ncbi.nlm.nih.gov/pmc/articles/PMC3825121/

El-Sherbiny GM1, E. S. (2011, 07). *The Effect of Commiphora molmol (Myrrh) in Treatment of Trichomoniasis vaginalis infection*. Retrieved 10 18, 2014, from Pubmed: http://www.ncbi.nlm.nih.gov/pubmed/22737515

Etman M1, A. M.-E. (2011, Jun). *Emulsions and rectal formulations containing myrrh essential oil for better patient compliance*. Retrieved 10 18, 2014, from Pubmed: http://www.ncbi.nlm.nih.gov/pubmed/22466245

Evans S1, D. N. (2010, 10 29). *The effect of a novel botanical agent TBS-101 on invasive prostate cancer in animal models*. Retrieved 10 18, 2014, from Pubmed: http://www.ncbi.nlm.nih.gov/pubmed/19846929

Fißler M, Q. A. (2014, 02 22). *A case series on the use of lavendula oil capsules in patients suffering from major depressive disorder and symptoms of psychomotor agitation, insomnia and anxiety*. Retrieved 10 16, 2014, from Pubmed.com: http://www.ncbi.nlm.nih.gov/pubmed/?term=lasea+MDD

Gómez-Rincón C, L. E. (2014). *Activity of tea tree (Melaleuca alternifolia) essential oil against L3 larvae of Anisakis simplex.* Retrieved 10 18, 2014, from Pubmed: http://www.ncbi.nlm.nih.gov/pubmed/24967378

Hosseini M1, G. R. (2011, 10 09). *Effects of different extracts of Rosa damascena on pentylenetetrazol-induced seizures in mice.* Retrieved 10 11, 2014, from Pubmed.com: http://www.ncbi.nlm.nih.gov/pubmed/22015194

How essential oils help the blood brain barrier. (2012). Retrieved 08 07, 2014, from Carlacohen.com: http://www.carlacohen.com/path-of-healing/young-living-education/blood-brain-barrierhow-the/

http://www.channel4.com/programmes/mummifying-alan-egypts-last-secret/videos/all/dr-stephen-buckley. (n.d.).

Ireland DJ1, G. S. (2012, 08). *Topically applied Melaleuca alternifolia (tea tree) oil causes direct anti-cancer cytotoxicity in subcutaneous tumour bearing mice.* Retrieved 10 18, 2014, from Pubmed: http://www.ncbi.nlm.nih.gov/pubmed/22727730

Jana Jones, T. F. (2014, 08). *Evidence for Prehistoric Origins of Egyptian Mummification in Late Neolithic Burials.* Retrieved 10 18, 2014, from Plosone:

http://www.plosone.org/article/info%3Adoi%2F10.1371%2Fjournal.pone.0103608

Kogiannou DA1, K. N. (2013, 11). *Herbal infusions; their phenolic profile, antioxidant and anti-inflammatory effects in HT29 and PC3 cells.* Retrieved 10 18, 2014, from Pubmed: http://www.ncbi.nlm.nih.gov/pubmed/23712099

Kolodziejczyk-Czepas J1, B. M.-M. (2014, 10 05). *Radical scavenging and antioxidant effects of Matricaria chamomilla polyphenolic-polysaccharide conjugates.* Retrieved 10 18, 2014, from Pubmed: http://www.ncbi.nlm.nih.gov/pubmed/25285848

Langhorst J1, F. A. (2014, 08 21). *Distinct kinetics in the frequency of peripheral CD4+ T cells in patients with ulcerative colitis experiencing a flare during treatment with mesalazine or with a herbal preparation of myrrh, chamomile, and coffee charcoal.* Retrieved 10 18, 2014, from Pubmed: http://www.ncbi.nlm.nih.gov/pubmed/25144293

Langhorst J1, F. A. (2014, 08 21). *Distinct kinetics in the frequency of peripheral CD4+ T cells in patients with ulcerative colitis experiencing a flare during treatment with mesalazine or with a herbal preparation of myrrh, chamomile, and coffee charcoal*. Retrieved 10 18, 2014, from Pubmed: http://www.ncbi.nlm.nih.gov/pubmed/25144293

Lee K1, L. J. (2014, 07 16). *Anti-biofilm, anti-hemolysis, and anti-virulence activities of black pepper, cananga, myrrh oils, and nerolidol against Staphylococcus aureus*. Retrieved 10 18, 2014, from Pubmed:
http://www.ncbi.nlm.nih.gov/pubmed/25027570

Li GH, Z. Q. (2013, 10). *Antiproliferative effect of cycloartane-type triterpenoid from myrrh against human prostate cancer cells*. Retrieved 10 18, 2014, from Pubmed:
http://www.ncbi.nlm.nih.gov/pubmed/24761675

Malik T1, S. P. (2011, 08 25). *Potentiation of antimicrobial activity of ciprofloxacin by Pelargonium graveolens essential oil against selected uropathogens*. Retrieved 10 18, 2014, from Pubmed:
http://www.ncbi.nlm.nih.gov/pubmed/?term=Ciprofloxicin+pelargonium

Manniche, L. (1989). *An Ancient Egyptian Herbal*. London: The British Museum Press.

Manniche, L. (1999). *Sacred Luxuries, Fragrance, Aromatherapy & Cosmetics in Ancient Egypt*. London: Opus Publishing.

McKay DL1, B. J. (2006, 07). *A review of the bioactivity and potential health benefits of chamomile tea (Matricaria recutita L.)*. Retrieved 10 18, 2014, from Pubmed: http://www.ncbi.nlm.nih.gov/pubmed/?term=camomile+matricaria+antiplatelets

Mohammadpour T, H. M. (2014, 06 29). *Protection against brain tissues oxidative damage as a possible mechanism for the beneficial effects of Rosa damascena hydroalcoholic extract on scopolamine induced memory impairment in rats*. Retrieved 10 11, 2014, from Pubmed.com: http://www.ncbi.nlm.nih.gov/pubmed/24974980

Nagai K1, N. A. (2014, 06 25). *Olfactory stimulatory with grapefruit and lavender oils change autonomic nerve activity and physiological function*. Retrieved 10 16, 2014, from Pubmed.com: http://www.ncbi.nlm.nih.gov/pubmed/25002406

P. Pommier, F. G. (2004). *Phase III Randomized Trial of Calendula Officinalis Compared With Trolamine for the Prevention of Acute Dermatitis During Irradiation for Breast*

Cancer. Retrieved 10 17, 2014, from Journal of Clinical Oncology: http://jco.ascopubs.org/content/22/8/1447.full

Press, T. (2011, 10 24). *Mummyfication: University of York chemist perfects art of Egyptian embalming*. Retrieved 10 18, 2014, from York Press: http://www.yorkpress.co.uk/features/features/9322267._I___m_the_only_woman_in_the_country_who___s_got_a_mummy_for_a_husband_/

Rafraf M1, Z. M.-J. (2014, 09 07). *Effectiveness of chamomile tea on glycemic control and serum lipid profile in patients with type 2 diabetes*. Retrieved 10 18, 2014, from Pubmed: http://www.ncbi.nlm.nih.gov/pubmed/25194428

Romero Mdel C1, V. A.-S.-M. (2012, 04 15). *Activity of Matricaria chamomilla essential oil against anisakiasis*. Retrieved 10 18, 2014, from Pubmed: http://www.ncbi.nlm.nih.gov/pubmed/22397992

Sachs, M. (1994). *Ayurveda Beauty Care*. Twin Lakes, USA: Lotus Press.

Santamaria M Jr1, P. K. (2014, 02). *Antimicrobial effect of Melaleuca alternifolia dental gel in orthodontic patients*. Retrieved 10 18, 2014, from Pubmed:

http://www.ncbi.nlm.nih.gov/pubmed/?term=Colgate++tea+tree

Saxena S1, U. V. (2012, 10). *Inhibitory effect of essential oils against Trichosporon ovoides causing Piedra Hair Infection.* Retrieved 10 18, 2014, from Pubmed: http://www.ncbi.nlm.nih.gov/pubmed/24031963

Sebai H1, J. M.-B. (2014, 03 14). *Antidiarrheal and antioxidant activities of chamomile (Matricaria recutita L.) decoction extract in rats.* Retrieved 10 18, 2014, from Pubmed: http://www.ncbi.nlm.nih.gov/pubmed/24463157

Sebai H1, J. M.-B. (2014, 03 14). *Antidiarrheal and antioxidant activities of chamomile (Matricaria recutita L.) decoction extract in rats.* Retrieved 10 18, 2014, from Pubmed: http://www.ncbi.nlm.nih.gov/pubmed/24463157

Sebai H1, S. S. (2014, 08 08). *Protective Effect of Lavandula stoechas and Rosmarinus officinalis Essential Oils Against Reproductive Damage and Oxidative Stress in Alloxan-Induced Diabetic Rats.* Retrieved 10 16, 2004, from Pubmed.com: http://www.ncbi.nlm.nih.gov/pubmed/25105335

Sharifi F1, S. M. (2014, 02 02). *Comparison of the effects of Matricaria chamomila (Chamomile) extract and mefenamic acid on the intensity of premenstrual syndrome.* Retrieved 10 18, 2014, from Pubmed: http://www.ncbi.nlm.nih.gov/pubmed/24439651

Sienkiewicz M1, P.-K. K. (2014, 08). *The antibacterial activity of geranium oil against Gram-negative bacteria isolated from difficult-to-heal wounds.* Retrieved 10 18, 2014, from Pubmed: http://www.ncbi.nlm.nih.gov/pubmed/24290961

Srivastava JK1, G. S. (2007, 11 07). *Antiproliferative and apoptotic effects of chamomile extract in various human cancer cells.* Retrieved 10 18, 2014, from Pubmed: http://www.ncbi.nlm.nih.gov/pubmed/17939735

Tabanca N1, W. M. (2013, 05 01). *Bioactivity-guided investigation of geranium essential oils as natural tick repellents.* Retrieved 10 18, 2014, from http://www.ncbi.nlm.nih.gov/pubmed/23528036

Tisserand, R. (1985). *The Art of Aromatherapy.* Saffron Waldron, Essex: The C W Daniel Co Ltd.

(2013). Cassia. In R. Tisserand, & Y. Rodney, *Essential OIl Safety: A Guide for Health Care Professionals* (pp. Kindle Locations 15361-15364)). Elsevier Health Sciences UK. Kindle Edition.

Tisserand, R., & Young, R. (.-1.-0. (2013). Agarwood. In *Essential Oil Safety: A Guide for Health Care Professionals* (pp. Kindle Locations 12825-12826)). Elsevier Health Sciences UK. Kindle Edition.

Tisserand, R., & Young, R. (.-1.-0. Anise. In *Essential Oil Safety: A Guide for Health Care Professionals* (pp. Kindle Locations 13160-13163). Elsevier Health Sciences UK. Kindle Edition. .

Tisserand, R., & Young, R. (.-1.-0. (2013). Benzoin. In R. Y. Robert Tisserand, *Essential Oil Safety: A Guide for Health Care Professionals* (pp. Kindle Locations 13983-13984). Elsevier Health Sciences UK. Kindle Edition.

Tisserand, R., & Young, R. (.-1.-0. Bergamot. In *Essential Oil Safety: A Guide for Health Care Professionals* (pp. Kindle Locations 14040-14043). Elsevier Health Sciences UK. Kindle Edition. .

Tisserand, R., & Young, R. (.-1.-0. Cajuput. In *Essential Oil Safety: A Guide for Health Care Professionals* (pp. Kindle Locations 14734-14735). Elsevier Health Sciences UK. Kindle Edition. .

(2013). Carrot Seed. In R. Tisserand, & R. (.-1.-0. Young, *Essential Oil Safety: A Guide for Health Care Professionals*

(Kindle Locations 15258-15259) (pp. Kindle Locations 15258-15259). Elsevier Health Sciences UK. Kindle Edition.

Tisserand, R., & Young, R. (.-1.-0. (2013). Catnip. In *Essential Oil Safety: A Guide for Health Care Professionals* (pp. Kindle Locations 15455-15457)). Elsevier Health Sciences UK. Kindle Edition.

Tisserand, R., & Young, R. (.-1.-0. (2013). Celery Seed. In *Essential Oil Safety: A Guide for Health Care Professionals* (pp. Kindle Locations 15718-15719). Elsevier Health Sciences UK. Kindle Edition.

Tisserand, R., & Young, R. (.-1.-0. Fennel. In *Essential Oil Safety: A Guide for Health Care Professionals* (pp. Kindle Locations 17700-17704). Elsevier Health Sciences UK. Kindle Edition.

Tisserand, R., & Young, R. (.-1.-0. Star Anise. In *Essential Oil Safety: A Guide for Health Care Professionals* (pp. (Kindle Locations 13227-13230)). Elsevier Health Sciences UK. Kindle Edition.

Tisserand, R., & Young, R. (2013). Angelica Root. In *Essential Oil Safety: A Guide for Health Care Professionals* (pp. Kindle

Locations 13049-13051). Elsevier Health Sciences UK. Kindle Edition. .

(2013). Cade. In R. Tisserand, & R. Young, *Essential Oil Safety: A Guide for Health Care Professionals* (pp. Kindle Location 14640-14713). Elsevier Health Sciences UK. Kindle Edition. .

(2013). Cinnamon Leaf. In R. Tisserand, & R. Young, *Essential Oil Safety: A Guide for Health Care Professionals* (pp. Kindle Locations 16175-16187). Elsevier Health Sciences UK. Kindle Edition. .

(2013). Clove Bud. In R. Tisserand, & R. Young, *Essential Oil Safety: A Guide for Health Care Professionals* (pp. Kindle Locations 16478-16479). Elsevier Health Sciences UK. Kindle Edition.

(2014). Holy Basil. In R. Tisserand, & R. Young, *Essential Oil Safety: A Guide for Health Care Professionals* (pp. Kindle Locations 13604-13607). Elsevier Health Sciences UK. Kindle Edition.

Tisserand, R., & Young, R. Lemongrass. In R. Tisserand, & R. Young, *Essential Oil Safety: A Guide for Health Care Professionals* (pp. Kindle Locations 20846-20849). Elsevier Health Sciences UK. Kindle Edition.

Tisserand, R., & Young, R. (2013). Wintergreen. In *Essential Oil Safety: A Guide for Health Care Professionals* (pp. Kindle Locations 28507-28511). Elsevier Health Sciences UK. Kindle Edition. .

Tomić M1, P. V.-P.-D. (2014, 05 28). *Antihyperalgesic and antiedematous activities of bisabolol-oxides-rich matricaria oil in a rat model of inflammation.* Retrieved 10 18, 2014, from Pubmed: http://www.ncbi.nlm.nih.gov/pubmed/23983133

Totilo, R. (2012). *The Art of Making Perfume.* Rebecca At The Well Foundation.

Totilo, R. (2013). *The Essential Oils of Ancient Scripture.* Rebecca at the Well Foundation.

Ueno-Iio T1, S. M. (2014, 06 05). *Lavender essential oil inhalation suppresses allergic airway inflammation and mucous cell hyperplasia in a murine model of asthma.* Retrieved 10 16, 2014, from Pubmed.com: http://www.ncbi.nlm.nih.gov/pubmed/24909715

Valnet, D. J. (1996). *The Practice of Aromatherapy.* Saffron Waldron, Essex: C W Daniel Company Ltd.

Viable quantitative PCR for assessing the response of Candida albicans to antifungal treatment. (2013, 1). Retrieved 10 18,

2014, from Pubmed: http://www.ncbi.nlm.nih.gov/pubmed/23132341

Worwood, V. A. (1993). *Aromantics*. Reading, Berks: Cox and Wyman.

Yap PS1, K. T. (2014, 02 14). *Membrane disruption and anti-quorum sensing effects of synergistic interaction between Lavandula angustifolia (lavender oil) in combination with antibiotic against plasmid-conferred multi-drug-resistant Escherichia coli.* Retrieved 10 16, 2014, from Pubmed.com: http://www.ncbi.nlm.nih.gov/pubmed/24779580

Zhao J1, K. S. (2014, 03 28). *Octulosonic acid derivatives from Roman chamomile (Chamaemelum nobile) with activities against inflammation and metabolic disorder.* Retrieved 10 18, 2014, from http://www.ncbi.nlm.nih.gov/pubmed/24471493

Zhuang SR1, C. H. (2012, 03 12). *Effects of a Chinese medical herbs complex on cellular immunity and toxicity-related conditions of breast cancer patients.* Retrieved 10 18, 2014, from Pubmed: http://www.ncbi.nlm.nih.gov/pubmed/21864416

Zu Y1, Y. H. (2010, 04 30). *Activities of ten essential oils towards Propionibacterium acnes and PC-3, A-549 and MCF-7 cancer cells*. Retrieved 10 18, 2014, from Pubmed: http://www.ncbi.nlm.nih.gov/pubmed/20657472

Disclaimer

by SEQ Legal

(1) Introduction

This disclaimer governs the use of this book. [By using this book, you accept this disclaimer in full. / We will ask you to agree to this disclaimer before you can access the book.]

(2) Credit

This disclaimer was created using an SEQ Legal template.

(3) No advice

The book contains information about aromatherapy and the use of essential oils. The information is not advice, and should not be treated as such.

[You must not rely on the information in the book as an alternative to qualified medical advice from a health professional. advice from an appropriately qualified professional. If you have any specific questions about any medical matter you should consult an appropriately qualified professional.]

[If you think you may be suffering from any medical condition you should seek immediate medical attention. You should never delay seeking medical advice, disregard medical advice, or discontinue medical treatment because of information in the book.]

(4)   No representations or warranties

To the maximum extent permitted by applicable law and subject to section 6 below, we exclude all representations, warranties, undertakings and guarantees relating to the book.

Without prejudice to the generality of the foregoing paragraph, we do not represent, warrant, undertake or guarantee:

> that the information in the book is correct, accurate, complete or non-misleading;

> that the use of the guidance in the book will lead to any particular outcome or result; or

> in particular, that by using the guidance in the book you will heal disease or work in any way as a cure for illness.

(5) Limitations and exclusions of liability

The limitations and exclusions of liability set out in this section and elsewhere in this disclaimer: are subject to section 6 below; and govern all liabilities arising under the disclaimer or in relation to the book, including liabilities arising in contract, in tort (including negligence) and for breach of statutory duty.

We will not be liable to you in respect of any losses arising out of any event or events beyond our reasonable control.

We will not be liable to you in respect of any business losses, including without limitation loss of or damage to profits, income, revenue, use, production, anticipated savings, business, contracts, commercial opportunities or goodwill.

We will not be liable to you in respect of any loss or corruption of any data, database or software.

We will not be liable to you in respect of any special, indirect or consequential loss or damage.

(6) Exceptions

Nothing in this disclaimer shall: limit or exclude our liability for death or personal injury resulting from negligence; limit or exclude our liability for fraud or fraudulent misrepresentation; limit any of our liabilities in any way that is not permitted under applicable law; or exclude any of our liabilities that may not be excluded under applicable law.

(7) Severability

If a section of this disclaimer is determined by any court or other competent authority to be unlawful and/or unenforceable, the other sections of this disclaimer continue in effect.

If any unlawful and/or unenforceable section would be lawful or enforceable if part of it were deleted, that part will be deemed to be deleted, and the rest of the section will continue in effect.

(8) Law and jurisdiction

This disclaimer will be governed by and construed in accordance with English law, and any disputes relating to this disclaimer will be subject to the exclusive jurisdiction of the courts of England and Wales.

(9) Our details

In this disclaimer, "we" means (and "us" and "our" refer to) [*Elizabeth Ashley* of [*Buildyourownreality.com 4, SY8 1LQ)*].

Printed in Great Britain
by Amazon